AMERICAN PSYCHIATRIC ASSOCIATION

BENJAMIN RUSH

1844

DIAGNOSTIC CRITERIA

FROM

DSM-III-R

Table of Contents

	Page
Introduction	v
Cautionary Statement	vii
DSM-III-R Classification	1
Use of This Manual	25

The Diagnostic Categories

Disorders Usually First Evident in Infancy, Childhood, or Adolescence	47
Organic Mental Syndromes and Disorders	77
Organic Mental Syndromes	77
Dementias Arising in the Senium and Presenium	84
Psychoactive Substance-induced Organic Mental Disorders	86
Organic Mental Disorders associated with Axis III physical disorders or conditions, or whose etiology is unknown	104
Psychoactive Substance Use Disorders	107
Schizophrenia	113
Delusional Disorder	119
Psychotic Disorders Not Elsewhere Classified	121
Mood Disorders	125
Anxiety Disorders	139
Somatoform Disorders	151
Dissociative Disorders	157

Sexual Disorders   161
Sleep Disorders   171
Factitious Disorders   177
Impulse Control Disorders Not Elsewhere
    Classified   179
Adjustment Disorder   183
Psychological Factors Affecting Physical
    Condition   187
Personality Disorders   189
V Codes for Conditions Not Attributable to a
    Mental Disorder That Are a Focus of
    Attention or Treatment   203
Additional Codes   209

Appendix A Proposed Diagnostic Categories
              Needing Further Study   211

Appendix B Decision Trees for Differential
              Diagnosis   219

Appendix C Alphabetic Listing of
              DSM-III-R Diagnoses   233

Appendix D Numeric Listing of
              DSM-III-R Codes   247

Abbreviated Symptom Index   261

Diagnostic Index   305

Introduction

One of the most important features of DSM-III-R is its provision of diagnostic criteria to improve the reliability of diagnostic judgments. With this approach, the clinician's task is twofold: to determine the presence or absence of specific clinical features, and then to use the criteria provided as guidelines for making the diagnosis. For quick reference, the clinician may wish to have available a small manual that contains only the classification, the diagnostic criteria, decision trees that aid in understanding the organization of the classification, an abbreviated symptom-based index, and alphabetic and numeric listings of the diagnoses and codes—hence, this Reference to the Diagnostic Criteria from DSM-III-R, which we affectionately call the "Mini-D."

Proper use of this manual requires familiarity with the description of the diagnostic categories and with the glossary of definitions of technical terms contained in DSM-III-R.

Robert L. Spitzer, M.D.
Chair, Work Group to Revise DSM-III

Janet B.W. Williams, D.S.W.
Text Editor

Cautionary Statement

The specified diagnostic criteria for each mental disorder are offered as guidelines for making diagnoses, since it has been demonstrated that the use of such criteria enhances agreement among clinicians and investigators. The proper use of these criteria requires specialized clinical training that provides both a body of knowledge and clinical skills.

These diagnostic criteria reflect a consensus of current formulations of evolving knowledge in our field but do not encompass all the conditions that may be legitimate objects of treatment or research efforts.

The purpose of DSM-III-R is to provide clear descriptions of diagnostic categories in order to enable clinicians and investigators to diagnose, communicate about, study, and treat the various mental disorders. It is to be understood that inclusion here, for clinical and research purposes, of a diagnostic category such as Pathological Gambling or Pedophilia does not imply that the condition meets legal or other nonmedical criteria for what constitutes mental disease, mental disorder, or mental disability. The clinical and scientific considerations involved in categorization of these conditions as mental disorders may not be wholly relevant to legal judgments, for example, that take into account such issues as individual responsibility, disability determination, and competency.

DSM-III-R Classification

DSM-III-R Classification:
Axes I and II Categories and Codes

All official DSM-III-R codes are included in ICD-9-CM. Codes followed by a * are used for more than one DSM-III-R diagnosis or sub-type in order to maintain compatibility with ICD-9-CM.

A long dash following a diagnostic term indicates the need for a fifth digit subtype or other qualifying term.

Numbers in parentheses are page numbers.

The term *specify* following the name of some diagnostic categories indicates qualifying terms that clinicians may wish to add in parentheses after the name of the disorder.

NOS = Not Otherwise Specified

The current severity of a disorder may be specified after the diagnosis as:

mild ⎱
moderate ⎬—— currently meets diagnostic criteria
severe ⎰

in partial remission
   (or residual state)
in complete remission

DISORDERS USUALLY FIRST EVIDENT IN INFANCY, CHILDHOOD, OR ADOLESCENCE

DEVELOPMENTAL DISORDERS

Note: These are coded on Axis II.

Mental Retardation (47)

317.00	Mild mental retardation
318.00	Moderate mental retardation
318.10	Severe mental retardation
318.20	Profound mental retardation
319.00	Unspecified mental retardation

Pervasive Developmental Disorders (49)

299.00	Autistic disorder
	Specify if childhood onset
299.80	Pervasive developmental disorder NOS

Specific Developmental Disorders (52)

Academic skills disorders (52)

315.10	Developmental arithmetic disorder
315.80	Developmental expressive writing disorder
315.00	Developmental reading disorder

Language and speech disorders (53)

315.39	Developmental articulation disorder
315.31*	Developmental expressive language disorder
315.31*	Developmental receptive language disorder

Motor skills disorder (55)

315.40	Developmental coordination disorder
315.90*	Specific developmental disorder NOS

Other Developmental Disorders (56)

315.90*   Developmental disorder NOS

Disruptive Behavior Disorders (56)

314.01   Attention-deficit hyperactivity disorder

           Conduct disorder,
312.20   group type
312.00   solitary aggressive type
312.90   undifferentiated type
313.81   Oppositional defiant disorder

Anxiety Disorders of Childhood or Adolescence (61)

309.21   Separation anxiety disorder
313.21   Avoidant disorder of childhood or adolescence
313.00   Overanxious disorder

Eating Disorders (63)

307.10   Anorexia nervosa
307.51   Bulimia nervosa
307.52   Pica
307.53   Rumination disorder of infancy
307.50   Eating disorder NOS

Gender Identity Disorders (65)

302.60   Gender identity disorder of childhood
302.50   Transsexualism
        Specify sexual history: asexual, homosexual, heterosexual, unspecified

302.85*   Gender identity disorder of adolescence
          or adulthood, nontranssexual type
              Specify sexual history: asexual, homo-
              sexual, heterosexual, unspecified
302.85*   Gender identity disorder NOS

Tic Disorders (68)

307.23   Tourette's disorder
307.22   Chronic motor or vocal tic disorder
307.21   Transient tic disorder
              Specify: single episode or recurrent
307.20   Tic disorder NOS

Elimination Disorders (70)

307.70   Functional encopresis
              Specify: primary or secondary type
307.60   Functional enuresis
              Specify: primary or secondary type
              Specify: nocturnal only, diurnal only,
              nocturnal and diurnal

Speech Disorders Not Elsewhere Classified (72)

307.00*   Cluttering
307.00*   Stuttering

**Other Disorders of Infancy, Childhood, or
Adolescence** (72)

313.23   Elective mutism
313.82   Identity disorder
313.89   Reactive attachment disorder of infancy or
          early childhood
307.30   Stereotypy/habit disorder
314.00   Undifferentiated attention-deficit disorder

ORGANIC MENTAL DISORDERS (77)

Dementias Arising in the Senium and Presenium (84)

Primary degenerative dementia of the Alzheimer type, senile onset

290.30	with delirium
290.20	with delusions
290.21	with depression
290.00*	uncomplicated

(Note: code 331.00 Alzheimer's disease on Axis III)

Code in fifth digit: 1 = with delirium, 2 = with delusions, 3 = with depression, 0* = uncomplicated.

290.1x	Primary degenerative dementia of the Alzheimer type, presenile onset, _____ (Note: code 331.00 Alzheimer's disease on Axis III)
290.4x	Multi-infarct dementia, _____
290.00*	Senile dementia NOS *Specify* etiology on Axis III if known
290.10*	Presenile dementia NOS *Specify* etiology on Axis III if known (e.g., Pick's disease, Jakob-Creutzfeldt disease)

Psychoactive Substance-Induced Organic Mental Disorders (86)

Alcohol (86)

303.00	intoxication
291.40	idiosyncratic intoxication

291.00   withdrawal delirium
291.30   hallucinosis
291.10   amnestic disorder
291.20   Dementia associated with alcoholism

Amphetamine or similarly acting
sympathomimetic (89)
305.70*   intoxication
292.00*   withdrawal
292.81*   delirium
292.11*   delusional disorder

Caffeine (91)
305.90*   intoxication

Cannabis (91)
305.20*   intoxication
292.11*   delusional disorder

Cocaine (92)
305.60*   intoxication
292.00*   withdrawal
292.81*   delirium
292.11*   delusional disorder

Hallucinogen (94)
305.30*   hallucinosis
292.11*   delusional disorder
292.84*   mood disorder
292.89*   Posthallucinogen perception disorder

Inhalant (96)
305.90*   intoxication

Nicotine (97)
292.00*   withdrawal

Opioid (97)
305.50*   intoxication
292.00*   withdrawal

Phencyclidine (PCP) or similarly acting arylcyclohexylamine (98)

305.90*	intoxication
292.81*	delirium
292.11*	delusional disorder
292.84*	mood disorder
292.90*	organic mental disorder NOS

Sedative, hypnotic, or anxiolytic (101)

305.40*	intoxication
292.00*	Uncomplicated sedative, hypnotic, or anxiolytic withdrawal
292.00*	withdrawal delirium
292.83*	amnestic disorder

Other or unspecified psychoactive substance (103)

305.90*	intoxication
292.00*	withdrawal
292.81*	delirium
292.82*	dementia
292.83*	amnestic disorder
292.11*	delusional disorder
292.12	hallucinosis
292.84*	mood disorder
292.89*	anxiety disorder
292.89*	personality disorder
292.90*	organic mental disorder NOS

Organic Mental Disorders associated with Axis III physical disorders or conditions, or whose etiology is unknown. (77)

293.00	Delirium (77)
294.10	Dementia (78)
294.00	Amnestic disorder (80)
293.81	Organic delusional disorder (81)
293.82	Organic hallucinosis (81)

293.83	Organic mood disorder (81)
	Specify: manic, depressed, mixed
294.80*	Organic anxiety disorder (82)
310.10	Organic personality disorder (82)
	Specify if explosive type
294.80*	Organic mental disorder NOS

PSYCHOACTIVE SUBSTANCE USE DISORDERS
(107)

Alcohol
303.90	dependence
305.00	abuse

Amphetamine or similarly acting
sympathomimetic
304.40	dependence
305.70*	abuse

Cannabis
304.30	dependence
305.20*	abuse

Cocaine
304.20	dependence
305.60*	abuse

Hallucingoen
304.50*	dependence
305.30*	abuse

Inhalant
304.60	dependence
305.90*	abuse

Nicotine
305.10	dependence

Opioid
304.00	dependence
305.50*	abuse

Phencyclidine (PCP) or similarly acting
arylcyclohexylamine
304.50* dependence
305.90* abuse

Sedative, hypnotic, or anxiolytic
304.10 dependence
305.40* abuse

304.90* Polysubstance dependence (110)
304.90* Psychoactive substance dependence NOS
305.90* Psychoactive substance abuse NOS

SCHIZOPHRENIA (113)

Code in fifth digit: 1 = subchronic, 2 = chronic,
3 = subchronic with acute exacerbation,
4 = chronic with acute exacerbation, 5 = in
remission, 0 = unspecified.

Schizophrenia
295.2x catatonic, _____
295.1x disorganized, _____
295.3x paranoid, _____
    Specify if stable type
295.9x undifferentiated, _____
295.6x residual, _____

Specify if late onset

DELUSIONAL (PARANOID) DISORDER (119)

297.10 Delusional (Paranoid) disorder

Specify type: erotomanic
        grandiose
        jealous
        persecutory
        somatic
        unspecified

PSYCHOTIC DISORDERS NOT ELSEWHERE CLASSIFIED (121)

298.80	Brief reactive psychosis
295.40	Schizophreniform disorder
	Specify: without good prognostic features or with good prognostic features
295.70	Schizoaffective disorder
	Specify: bipolar type or depressive type
297.30	Induced psychotic disorder
298.90	Psychotic disorder NOS (Atypical psychosis)

MOOD DISORDERS (125)

Code current state of Major Depression and Bipolar Disorder in fifth digit:

1 = mild
2 = moderate
3 = severe, without psychotic features
4 = with psychotic features (*specify* mood-congruent or mood-incongruent)
5 = in partial remission
6 = in full remission
0 = unspecified

For major depressive episodes, *specify* if chronic and *specify* if melancholic type.

For Bipolar Disorder, Bipolar Disorder NOS, Recurrent Major Depression, and Depressive Disorder NOS, *specify* if seasonal pattern.

Bipolar Disorders (132)

	Bipolar disorder
296.6x	mixed, _____
296.4x	manic, _____
296.5x	depressed, _____

301.13   Cyclothymia
296.70   Bipolar disorder NOS

Depressive Disorders (135)

       Major Depression
296.2x   single episode, _____
296.3x   recurrent, _____
300.40   Dysthymia (or Depressive neurosis)
       Specify: primary or secondary type
       Specify: early or late onset
311.00   Depressive disorder NOS

ANXIETY DISORDERS (or Anxiety and Phobic Neuroses) (139)

       Panic disorder
300.21   with agoraphobia
       Specify current severity of agoraphobic avoidance
       Specify current severity of panic attacks
300.01   without agoraphobia
       Specify: current severity of panic attacks
300.22   Agoraphobia without history of panic disorder
       Specify with or without limited symptom attacks
300.23   Social phobia
       Specify if generalized type
300.29   Simple phobia
300.30   Obsessive compulsive disorder (or Obsessive compulsive neurosis)
309.89   Post-traumatic stress disorder
       Specify if delayed onset
300.02   Generalized anxiety disorder
300.00   Anxiety disorder NOS

SOMATOFORM DISORDERS (151)

300.70*	Body dysmorphic disorder
300.11	Conversion disorder (or Hysterical neurosis, conversion type)
	Specify: single episode or recurrent
300.70*	Hypochondriasis (or Hypochondriacal neurosis)
300.81	Somatization disorder
307.80	Somatoform pain disorder
300.70*	Undifferentiated somatoform disorder
300.70*	Somatoform disorder NOS

DISSOCIATIVE DISORDERS (or Hysterical Neuroses, Dissociative Type) (157)

300.14	Multiple personality disorder
300.13	Psychogenic fugue
300.12	Psychogenic amnesia
300.60	Depersonalization disorder (or Depersonalization neurosis)
300.15	Dissociative disorder NOS

SEXUAL DISORDERS (161)

Paraphilias (161)

302.40	Exhibitionism
302.81	Fetishism
302.89	Frotteurism
302.20	Pedophilia
	Specify: same sex, opposite sex, same and opposite sex
	Specify if limited to incest
	Specify: exclusive type or nonexclusive type
302.83	Sexual masochism
302.84	Sexual sadism

302.30   Transvestic fetishism
302.82   Voyeurism
302.90*   Paraphilia NOS

Sexual Dysfunctions (164)

Specify: psychogenic only, or psychogenic and bio-
    genic (Note: If biogenic only, code on Axis III)
Specify: lifelong or acquired
Specify: generalized or situational

Sexual desire disorders
302.71   Hypoactive sexual desire disorder
302.79   Sexual aversion disorder

Sexual arousal disorders
302.72*   Female sexual arousal disorder
302.72*   Male erectile disorder

Orgasm disorders
302.73   Inhibited female orgasm
302.74   Inhibited male orgasm
302.75   Premature ejaculation

Sexual pain disorders
302.76   Dyspareunia
306.51   Vaginismus

302.70   Sexual dysfunction NOS

Other Sexual Disorders (168)

302.90*   Sexual disorder NOS

SLEEP DISORDERS (171)

Dyssomnias (171)

Insomnia disorder
307.42*   related to another mental disorder (non-
          organic)

780.50*	related to known organic factor
307.42*	Primary insomnia

Hypersomnia disorder
307.44	related to another mental disorder (non-organic)
780.50*	related to a known organic factor
780.54	Primary hypersomnia
307.45	Sleep-wake schedule disorder

Specify: advanced or delayed phase type, disorganized type, frequently changing type

Other dyssomnias
| 307.40* | Dyssomnia NOS |

Parasomnias (175)

307.47	Dream anxiety disorder (Nightmare disorder)
307.46*	Sleep terror disorder
307.46*	Sleepwalking disorder
307.40*	Parasomnia NOS

FACTITIOUS DISORDERS (177)

Factitious disorder
301.51	with physical symptoms
300.16	with psychological symptoms
300.19	Factitious disorder NOS

IMPULSE CONTROL DISORDERS NOT ELSEWHERE CLASSIFIED (179)

312.34	Intermittent explosive disorder
312.32	Kleptomania
312.31	Pathological gambling
312.33	Pyromania
312.39*	Trichotillomania
312.39*	Impulse control disorder NOS

ADJUSTMENT DISORDER (183)

	Adjustment disorder
309.24	with anxious mood
309.00	with depressed mood
309.30	with disturbance of conduct
309.40	with mixed disturbance of emotions and conduct
309.28	with mixed emotional features
309.82	with physical complaints
309.83	with withdrawal
309.23	with work (or academic) inhibition
309.90	Adjustment disorder NOS

PSYCHOLOGICAL FACTORS AFFECTING PHYSICAL CONDITION (187)

316.00	Psychological factors affecting physical condition
	Specify physical condition on Axis III

PERSONALITY DISORDERS (189)

Note: These are coded on Axis II.

Cluster A (189)

301.00	Paranoid
301.20	Schizoid
301.22	Schizotypal

Cluster B (192)

301.70	Antisocial
301.83	Borderline
301.50	Histrionic
301.81	Narcissistic

Cluster C (197)

301.82	Avoidant
301.60	Dependent
301.40	Obsessive compulsive
301.84	Passive aggressive
301.90	Personality disorder NOS

V CODES FOR CONDITIONS NOT ATTRIBUTABLE TO A MENTAL DISORDER THAT ARE A FOCUS OF ATTENTION OR TREATMENT (203)

V62.30	Academic problem
V71.01	Adult antisocial behavior

V40.00	Borderline intellectual functioning (Note: This is coded on Axis II.)

V71.02	Childhood or adolescent antisocial behavior
V65.20	Malingering
V61.10	Marital problem
V15.81	Noncompliance with medical treatment
V62.20	Occupational problem
V61.20	Parent-child problem
V62.81	Other interpersonal problem
V61.80	Other specified family circumstances
V62.89	Phase of life problem or other life circumstance problem
V62.82	Uncomplicated bereavement

ADDITIONAL CODES (209)

300.90	Unspecified mental disorder (non-psychotic)
V71.09*	No diagnosis or condition on Axis I

799.90*   Diagnosis or condition deferred on Axis I

V71.09*	No diagnosis or condition on Axis II
799.90*	Diagnosis or condition deferred on Axis II

MULTIAXIAL SYSTEM

Axis I   Clinical Syndromes
         V Codes

Axis II   Developmental Disorders
         Personality Disorders

Axis III Physical Disorders and Conditions

Axis IV   Severity of Psychosocial Stressors

Axis V   Global Assessment of Functioning

Severity of Psychosocial Stressors Scale: Adults

See p. 33 for instructions on how to use this scale.

Code	Term	Examples of stressors	
		Acute events	Enduring circumstances
1	None	No acute events that may be relevant to the disorder	No enduring circumstances that may be relevant to the disorder
2	Mild	Broke up with boyfriend or girlfriend; started or graduated from school; child left home	Family arguments; job dissatisfaction; residence in high-crime neighborhood
3	Moderate	Marriage; marital separation; loss of job; retirement; miscarriage	Marital discord; serious financial problems; trouble with boss; being a single parent
4	Severe	Divorce; birth of first child	Unemployment; poverty
5	Extreme	Death of spouse; serious physical illness diagnosed; victim of rape	Serious chronic illness in self or child; ongoing physical or sexual abuse
6	Catastrophic	Death of child; suicide of spouse; devastating natural disaster	Captivity as hostage; concentration camp experience
0	Inadequate information, or no change in condition		

20

Severity of Psychosocial Stressors Scale: Children and Adolescents
See p. 33 for instructions on how to use this scale.

Code	Term	Examples of stressors	
		Acute events	**Enduring circumstances**
1	None	No acute events that may be relevant to the disorder	No enduring circumstances that may be relevant to the disorder
2	Mild	Broke up with boyfriend or girlfriend; change of school	Overcrowded living quarters; family arguments
3	Moderate	Expelled from school; birth of sibling	Chronic disabling illness in parent; chronic parental discord
4	Severe	Divorce of parents; unwanted pregnancy; arrest	Harsh or rejecting parents; chronic life-threatening illness in parent; multiple foster home placements
5	Extreme	Sexual or physical abuse; death of a parent	Recurrent sexual or physical abuse
6	Catastrophic	Death of both parents	Chronic life-threatening illness
0	Inadequate information, or no change in condition		

21

Global Assessment of Functioning Scale (GAF Scale)

Consider psychological, social, and occupational functioning on a hypothetical continuum of mental health–illness. Do not include impairment in functioning due to physical (or environmental) limitations. See p. 37 for instructions on how to use this scale.

Note: Use intermediate codes when appropriate, e.g., 45, 68, 72.

Code

90 — **Absent or minimal symptoms** (e.g., mild anxiety before an exam), **good functioning in all areas, interested and involved in a wide range of activities, socially effective, generally satisfied with life, no more than everyday problems or concerns** (e.g., an occasional argument with family members).

81 —

80 — **If symptoms are present, they are transient and expectable reactions to psychosocial stressors** (e.g., difficulty concentrating after family argument); **no more than slight impairment in social, occupational, or school functioning** (e.g., temporarily falling behind in school work).

71 —

70 — **Some mild symptoms** (e.g., depressed mood and mild insomnia) **OR some difficulty in social, occupational, or school functioning** (e.g., occasional truancy, or theft within the household), **but generally functioning pretty well, has some meaningful interpersonal relationships.**

61 —

60 — **Moderate symptoms** (e.g., flat affect and circumstantial speech, occasional panic attacks) **OR moderate difficulty in social, occupational, or school functioning** (e.g., few friends, conflicts with co-workers).

51 —

22

50

41

Serious symptoms (e.g., suicidal ideation, severe obsessional rituals, frequent shoplifting) **OR any serious impairment in social, occupational, or school functioning** (e.g., no friends, unable to keep a job).

40

31

Some impairment in reality testing or communication (e.g., speech is at times illogical, obscure, or irrelevant) **OR major impairment in several areas, such as work or school, family relations, judgment, thinking, or mood** (e.g., depressed man avoids friends, neglects family, and is unable to work; child frequently beats up younger children, is defiant at home, and is failing at school).

30

21

Behavior is considerably influenced by delusions or hallucinations OR serious impairment in communication or judgment (e.g., sometimes incoherent, acts grossly inappropriately, suicidal preoccupation) **OR inability to function in almost all areas** (e.g., stays in bed all day; no job, home, or friends).

20

11

Some danger of hurting self or others (e.g., suicide attempts without clear expectation of death, frequently violent, manic excitement) **OR occasionally fails to maintain minimal personal hygiene** (e.g., smears feces) **OR gross impairment in communication** (e.g., largely incoherent or mute).

10

1

Persistent danger of severely hurting self or others (e.g., recurrent violence) **OR persistent inability to maintain minimal personal hygiene OR serious suicidal act with clear expectation of death.**

Use of This Manual

Use of This Manual

This chapter includes a discussion of the following:

MULTIAXIAL EVALUATION, p. 27
   Axes I and II, p. 28
   Multiple diagnoses within Axes I and II, p. 29
   Axis II and description of personality features, p. 30
   Principal diagnosis, p. 30
   Provisional diagnosis, p. 31
   Levels of diagnostic certainty, p. 32
   Axis III, p. 33
   Axis IV, p. 33
   Axis V, p. 37
   Examples of how to record the results of a multi-axial evaluation, p. 38
EXPLANATION OF COMMONLY USED TERMS AND PHRASES, p. 39
SPECIFYING CURRENT SEVERITY OF DISORDER, p. 41

MULTIAXIAL EVALUATION

A multiaxial evaluation requires that every case be assessed on several "axes," each of which refers to a different class of information. In order for the system to have maximal clinical usefulness, there must be a limited number of axes; there are five in the DSM-III-R multiaxial classification. The first three axes constitute the official diagnostic assessment.

Use of the DSM-III-R multiaxial system ensures that attention is given to certain types of disorders, aspects of the environment, and areas of functioning that might be overlooked if the focus were on assessing a single presenting problem. Each person is evaluated on each of these axes:

Axis I   Clinical Syndromes and V Codes
Axis II   Developmental Disorders and Personality Disorders
Axis III   Physical Disorders and Conditions
Axis IV   Severity of Psychosocial Stressors
Axis V   Global Assessment of Functioning

Axes IV and V are available for use in special clinical and research settings; they provide information that supplements the official DSM-III-R diagnoses (on Axes I, II, and III) and that may be useful for planning treatment and predicting outcome.

Axes I and II. Mental Disorders and V Codes

Axes I and II constitute the entire classification of mental disorders plus V Codes (Conditions Not Attributable to a Mental Disorder That Are a Focus of Attention or Treatment). The disorders listed on Axis II, Developmental Disorders and Personality Disorders, generally begin in childhood or adolescence and persist in a stable form (without periods of remission or exacerbation) into adult life. With only a few exceptions (e.g., the Gender Identity Disorders and Paraphilias), these features are not characteristic of the Axis I disorders. The separation between Axis I and Axis II ensures that in the evaluation of adults, consideration is given to the possible presence of Personality Disorders that may be overlooked when attention is directed to the usually more florid Axis I disorder. The Axis I–Axis II distinction in evaluating children emphasizes the need to consider disorders involving the development of cognitive, social, and motor skills.

In many instances there will be a disorder on both axes. For example, an adult may have Major Depression noted on Axis I and Obsessive Compulsive Personality Disorder on Axis II, or a child may have Conduct Disorder noted on Axis I and Developmental Language Disorder on Axis II. In other instances there may be no disorder on Axis I, the reason for seeking treatment being limited to a condition noted on Axis II. In this latter case, the clinician should write: *Axis I:* V71.09 No diagnosis or condition on Axis I, or one of the Conditions Not Attributable to a Mental Disorder should be recorded. On the other hand, if a disorder is noted on Axis I but there is no evidence of an Axis II disorder, the clinician should write: *Axis II:* V71.09 No diagnosis on Axis II.

Multiple diagnoses within Axes I and II

On both Axes I and II, multiple diagnoses should be made when necessary to describe the current condition. This applies particularly to Axis I, on which, for example, a person may have both a Psychoactive Substance Use Disorder and a Mood Disorder. It is also possible to have multiple diagnoses within the same class. For example, it is possible to have several Psychoactive Substance Use Disorders or, in the class of Mood Disorders, it is possible to have Major Depression superimposed on Dysthymia or Bipolar Disorder superimposed on Cyclothymia. In other classes, such as Schizophrenia, however, each of the types is mutually exclusive.

Within Axis II, the diagnosis of multiple Specific Developmental Disorders is common. For some adults the persistence of a Specific Developmental Disorder and the presence of a Personality Disorder may require that both be noted on Axis II. Usually, a single Personality Disorder will be noted; but when the person meets the criteria for more than one, all should be recorded.

Axis II and description of personality features

Axis II can be used to indicate specific personality traits or the habitual use of particular defense mechanisms (see Glossary for definitions). This can be done when no Personality Disorder exists or to supplement a Personality Disorder diagnosis. (Code numbers are not used when personality traits are noted, since a code number indicates a Personality Disorder.)

Examples:

Axis II: 301.40   Obsessive Compulsive Personality
                  Disorder with paranoid traits
Axis II: V71.09   No diagnosis on Axis II but massive
                  denial of Axis III disorder (juvenile
                  diabetes)

Principal diagnosis

When a person receives more than one diagnosis, the *principal* diagnosis is the condition that was chiefly responsible for occasioning the evaluation or admission to clinical care. In most cases this condition will be the main focus of attention or treatment. The principal diagnosis may be an Axis I or an Axis II diagnosis; but when an Axis II diagnosis is the principal diagnosis, the Axis II entry should be followed by the phrase "(Principal diagnosis)."

Example:

Axis I: 303.90 Alcohol Dependence
Axis II: 301.70 Antisocial Personality Disorder
                 (Principal diagnosis)

When a person has both an Axis I and an Axis II diagnosis, the principal diagnosis will be assumed to be on Axis I unless the Axis II diagnosis is followed by the qualifying phrase "(Principal diagnosis)."

When multiple diagnoses are made on either Axis I or Axis II, they should be listed within each axis in the order of focus of attention or treatment. For example, if a person with Schizophrenia, Paranoid Type, Chronic, comes to an emergency room for treatment of Alcohol Intoxication, the diagnosis should be listed:

Axis I: 303.00 Alcohol Intoxication
         295.32 Schizophrenia, Paranoid Type,
                 Chronic

Provisional diagnosis

In some instances not enough information will be available to make a firm diagnosis. The clinician may wish to indicate a significant degree of diagnostic uncertainty by writing "(Provisional)" following the diagnosis—e.g., Schizophreniform Disorder (Provisional, rule out Organic Delusional Disorder).

Levels of diagnostic certainty

The following table indicates the various ways in which a clinician may indicate diagnostic uncertainty:

Term	Examples of clinical situations
V Codes (for Conditions Not Attributable to a Mental Disorder That Are a Focus of Attention or Treatment)	Insufficient information to know whether or not a presenting problem is attributable to a mental disorder, e.g., Academic Problem; Adult Antisocial Behavior.
799.90 Diagnosis or Condition Deferred on Axis I	Information inadequate to make any diagnostic judgment about an Axis I diagnosis or condition.
799.90 Diagnosis Deferred on Axis II	Same for an Axis II diagnosis.
300.90 Unspecified Mental Disorder (nonpsychotic)	Enough information available to rule out a psychotic disorder, but further specification is not possible.
298.90 Psychotic Disorder Not Otherwise Specified	Enough information available to determine the presence of a psychotic disorder, but further specification is not possible.
(Class of disorder) Not Otherwise Specified	Enough information available to indicate the class of disorder that is present, but further specification is not possible, because either there is not sufficient information to make a more specific diagnosis, or the clinical features of the disorder do not meet the criteria for any of the specific categories in that class, e.g., Depressive Disorder Not Otherwise Specified.
Specific diagnosis (Provisional)	Enough information available to make a "working" diagnosis, but the clinician wishes to indicate a significant degree of diagnostic uncertainty, e.g., Schizophreniform Disorder (Provisional).

Axis III. Physical Disorders and Conditions

Axis III permits the clinician to indicate any current physical disorder or condition that is potentially relevant to the understanding or management of the case. These are the conditions listed outside the mental disorders section of ICD-9-CM. In some instances the condition may be etiologically significant (e.g., a neurologic disorder associated with Dementia); in other instances the physical disorder may not be etiologic, but important in the overall management of the case (e.g., diabetes in a child with Conduct Disorder). In yet other instances, the clinician may wish to note significant associated physical findings, such as "soft neurologic signs." Multiple diagnoses are permitted.

Axis IV. Severity of Psychosocial Stressors

Axis IV provides a scale, the Severity of Psychosocial Stressors Scale (see pp. 20 and 21), for coding the overall severity of a psychosocial stressor or multiple psychosocial stressors that have occurred in the year preceding the current evaluation and that may have contributed to any of the following:

(1) development of a new mental disorder,
(2) recurrence of a prior mental disorder,
(3) exacerbation of an already existing mental disorder (e.g., divorce occurring during a Major Depressive Episode, or during the course of chronic Schizophrenia).

(Note: Post-traumatic Stress Disorder is an exception to the requirement that the stressor has occurred within a year before the evaluation.) The current disorder that is related to the psychosocial stressor may be either a clinical syndrome, coded on Axis I, or an exacerbation of a Personality or Developmental Disorder, coded on Axis II. In some instances the stressor is anticipation of a future event, e.g., imminent retirement.

Although a stressor frequently plays a precipitating role in a disorder, it may also be a consequence of the person's psychopathology—e.g., Alcohol Dependence may lead to marital problems and divorce, which can then become stressors contributing to the development of a Major Depressive Episode.

Rating the severity of the stressor. The rating of the severity of the stressor should be based on the clinician's assessment of the stress an "average" person in similar circumstances and with similar sociocultural values would experience from the particular psychosocial stressor(s). This judgment involves consideration of the following: the amount of change in the person's life caused by the stressor, the degree to which the event is desired and under the person's control, and the number of stressors. For example, a planned pregnancy is usually less stressful than an unwanted pregnancy. Even though a specific stressor may have greater impact on a person who is especially vulnerable or has certain internal conflicts, the rating should be based on the severity of the stressor itself, not on the person's vulnerability to the particular stressor. If a vulnerability to stress exists, it will frequently be due to a mental disorder that is coded on Axis I or II.

The specific psychosocial stressor(s) should be noted and further specified as either:

predominantly acute events (duration less than six months)

predominantly enduring circumstances (duration greater than six months).

Examples of predominantly acute events are entering a new school or beginning a new job, having an accident, and death of a loved one. Examples of predominantly enduring circumstances are chronic marital or parental discord, and persistent and harsh parental discipline. The distinction between these two types of stressors may be important in formulating a treatment plan that includes attempts to remove the psychosocial stressor(s) or to help the person cope with it (them). Furthermore, there is evidence that predominantly enduring psychosocial stressors are more likely to predispose children to develop mental disorders than predominantly acute events.

In evaluating the stressors that may have contributed to the development of the current episode of illness, more than one may be judged to be relevant, but rarely should more than the four most severe be recorded. When more than one stressor is present, the severity rating will generally be that of the most severe stressor. However, in the case of multiple severe or extreme stressors, a higher rating should be considered. Each of the stressors should be noted and listed in the order of their importance.

Separate examples are given below for adults and for children and adolescents. These may be used as general guides for making the severity rating, the context in which the stressor(s) occurs being taken into account.

The code "0" should be used either when there is inadequate information about the presence or absence of psychosocial stressors to make a more definitive rating, or when the use of this axis is not appropriate because there has been no change in the person's condition (e.g., the person is being reevaluated after several months in the hospital because of a change of therapists).

Types of psychosocial stressors to be considered. To ascertain etiologically significant psychosocial stressors, the following areas may be considered:

Conjugal (marital and nonmarital): e.g., engagement, marriage, discord, separation, death of spouse.

Parenting: e.g., becoming a parent, friction with child, illness of child.

Other interpersonal: problems with one's friends, neighbors, associates, or nonconjugal family members, e.g., illness of best friend, discordant relationship with boss.

Occupational: includes work, school, homemaking, e.g., unemployment, retirement, school problems.

Living circumstances: e.g., change in residence, threat to personal safety, immigration.

Financial: e.g., inadequate finances, change in financial status.

Legal: e.g., arrest, imprisonment, lawsuit, or trial.

Developmental: phases of the life cycle, e.g., puberty, transition to adult status, menopause, "becoming 50."

Physical illness or injury: e.g., illness, accident, surgery, abortion. (_Note:_ A physical disorder is listed on Axis III whenever it is related to the development or management of an Axis I or II disorder. A physical disorder can also be a psychosocial stressor if its impact is due to its meaning to the individual, in which case it would be listed on both Axis III and Axis IV.)

Other psychosocial stressors: e.g., natural or man-made disaster, persecution, unwanted pregnancy, out-of-wedlock birth, rape.

Family factors (children and adolescents): In addition to the above, for children and adolescents the following stressors may be considered: cold, hostile, intrusive, abusive, conflictual, or confusingly inconsistent relationship between parents or toward child;

physical or mental illness in a family member; lack of parental guidance or excessively harsh or inconsistent parental control; insufficient, excessive, or confusing social or cognitive stimulation; anomalous family situation, e.g., complex or inconsistent parental custody and visitation arrangements; foster family; institutional rearing; loss of nuclear family members.

Axis V. Global Assessment of Functioning

Axis V permits the clinician to indicate his or her overall judgment of a person's psychological, social, and occupational functioning on a scale, the Global Assessment of Functioning Scale (GAF Scale),[1] that assesses mental health–illness. This scale appears on p. 22-23. Ratings on the GAF Scale should be made for two time periods:

(1) Current—the level of functioning at the time of the evaluation.
(2) Past year—the highest level of functioning for at least a few months during the past year. For children and adolescents, this should include at least a month during the school year.

Ratings of current functioning will generally reflect the current need for treatment or care. Ratings of highest level of functioning during the past year frequently will have prognostic significance, because usually a person returns to his or her previous level of functioning after an episode of illness.

---

[1] The GAF Scale is a revision of the GAS (Endicott J, Spitzer RL, Fleiss J, et al: The Global Assessment Scale: A procedure for measuring overall severity of psychiatric disturbance. *Archives of General Psychiatry* 33:766-771, 1976) and the CGAS (Shaffer D, Gould MS, Brasic J, et al: Children's Global Assessment Scale [CGAS]. *Archives of General Psychiatry* 40:1228-1231, 1983), which are revisions of the Health-Sickness Rating Scale (Luborsky L: Clinicians' judgments of mental health. *Archives of General Psychiatry* 7:407-417, 1962).

Examples of How To Record the Results of a DSM-III-R Multiaxial Evaluation

Example 1

Axis I:	296.23	Major Depression, Single Episode, Severe, without Psychotic Features
	303.90	Alcohol Dependence
Axis II:	301.60	Dependent Personality Disorder (Provisional, rule out Borderline Personality Disorder)

Axis III: Alcoholic cirrhosis of liver

Axis IV: Psychosocial stressors: anticipated retirement and change in residence, with loss of contact with friends
Severity: 4—Moderate (predominantly enduring circumstances)

Axis V: Current GAF: 44
Highest GAF past year: 55

Example 2

Axis I:	309.24	Adjustment Disorder with Anxious Mood
Axis II:	V71.09	No diagnosis on Axis II

Axis III: None

Axis IV: Psychosocial stressors: Change of school
Severity: 2—Mild (acute event)

Axis V: Current GAF: 70
Highest GAF past year: 85

Example 3

Axis I: 295.94   Schizophrenia, Undifferentiated Type, Chronic with Acute
Exacerbation

Axis II: V71.09   No diagnosis on Axis II

V40.00   Borderline Intellectual Functioning (Provisional)

Axis III: Late effects of viral encephalitis

Axis IV: Psychosocial stressors: death of mother
Severity: 6—Extreme (acute event)

Axis V: Current GAF: 28
Highest GAF past year: 40

EXPLANATION OF COMMONLY USED TERMS AND PHRASES

It cannot be established that an organic factor initiated and maintained the disturbance. This phrase is
used for certain diagnoses to indicate that the diagnosis is made only when, after an appropriate evaluation, the clinician cannot identify an organic factor
that is believed to have initiated *and* maintained the
disturbance. In some cases, the presence of an
etiologic organic factor can be established from the
history alone. In other cases, physical examination or
laboratory tests are necessary. For example, when a
person presents with symptoms characteristic of
Schizophrenia, the diagnosis can be made only when
the clinician concludes, after an appropriate evaluation, that no organic factor (such as a psychoactive
substance or a brain tumor) can be established to
have initiated and maintained the disturbance.

It should be noted that the organic factor must not only have initiated the disturbance but be responsible for *maintaining* the disturbance as well. For example, the diagnosis of Panic Disorder would still be appropriate in a situation in which the onset of the panic attacks was triggered by the use of cannabis, provided the panic attacks persisted for a significant period of time, such as one month, after use of the cannabis had stopped.

If a particular diagnosis is excluded because an organic factor that initiated and maintained the disturbance can be established, then the corresponding Organic Mental Disorder should be diagnosed. For example, if the diagnosis of Schizophrenia was excluded because of use of amphetamines, the diagnosis of an Organic Delusional Disorder should be made; if the diagnosis of a Major Depression was excluded because of a brain tumor, the diagnosis of an Organic Mood Disorder should be made.

The phrase *organic factor* is difficult to define precisely. However, in this context it refers to two major categories: (1) identifiable **exogenous** physical factors that affect the central nervous system, such as pharmacologic agents, infections, and trauma, and (2) identifiable **endogenous** factors, such as structural brain disease or metabolic disturbance. Genetically transmitted vulnerability and nonspecific abnormalities of central nervous system structure and function (including endocrinologic abnormalities) are generally **not** included as an organic factor in this context; these are present in only some people with the disorder, are present in some people without the disorder, and may be only associated features of the disorder, unrelated to the basic pathophysiologic process of the disturbance.

The fact that certain diagnoses are made only when an organic factor cannot be identified does not imply the absence of a fundamental biologic disturbance in these disorders. It should be understood that when we know more about the biologic mechanisms involved in such disorders as Schizophrenia, Bipolar Disorder, and Major Depression, we may be able to identify specific organic factors that are responsible for initiating and maintaining these disorders.

Occurrence is not exclusively during the course of [disorder]. This phrase is used in certain exclusion criteria to indicate that the diagnosis of the disorder being defined is not made if its defining symptoms or features have been present only when the other disorder was also present. For example, an exclusion criterion for Hypoactive Sexual Desire Disorder is "Occurrence is not exclusively during the course of a Major Depressive Episode," which means that if the lack of sexual desire was present only during a Major Depressive Episode, the additional diagnosis of Hypoactive Sexual Desire Disorder would not be made.

Not Otherwise Specified (NOS). This expression is used to indicate a category within a class of disorders that is residual to the specific categories in that class, although it is recognized that in some settings the category may actually be more common than any of the specific disorders in that particular class.

Physical disorders. The term *physical disorders* is used to refer to any disorder listed in ICD-9-CM outside the chapter on mental disorders.

SPECIFYING CURRENT SEVERITY OF DISORDER

The current severity of a disorder may be specified, following the diagnosis, by the following terms (in

parentheses): mild, moderate, severe, in partial remission (or residual state), in full remission.

Examples: Social Phobia (severe)
Alcohol Dependence (in full remission)
Attention-deficit Hyperactivity Disorder
(residual state)

"Mild," "moderate," and "severe" should be used
to indicate the severity of the current disorder (or
provisional disorder) at the time of the evaluation
when all of the diagnostic criteria are met. The distinction among mild, moderate, and severe should take
into account the number and intensity of the signs
and symptoms of the disorder and any resulting impairment in occupational or social functioning. For
the following disorders, specific criteria for levels of
severity are provided.

Attention-deficit Hyperactivity Disorder (p. 57)
Conduct Disorder (p. 59)
Oppositional Defiant Disorder (p. 60)
Dementia (p. 80)
Psychoactive Substance Dependence Disorders
(p. 108)
Manic episode (p. 126)
Major depressive episode (p. 129)
Panic Disorder with Agoraphobia (p. 141)
Paraphilias (p. 161)

For all the other disorders, the following guidelines
may be used:

Mild: Few, if any, symptoms in excess of those required to make the diagnosis **and** symptoms result in
only minor impairment in occupational functioning or
in usual social activities or relationships with others.

Moderate: Symptoms or functional impairment between "mild" and "severe."

Severe: Several symptoms in excess of those required to make the diagnosis **and** symptoms markedly interfere with occupational functioning or with usual social activities or relationships with others.

In Partial Remission or **Residual State:** The full criteria for the disorder were previously met, but currently only some of the symptoms or signs of the illness are present. *In partial remission* should be used when there is the expectation that the person will completely recover (or have a complete remission) within the next few years, as, for example, in the case of a Major Depressive Episode. *Residual state* should be used when there is little expectation of a complete remission or recovery within the next few years, as, for example, in the case of Autistic Disorder or Attention-deficit Hyperactivity Disorder. (*Residual state* should not be used with Schizophrenia, since by tradition there is a specific residual type of Schizophrenia.) In some cases the distinction between *in partial remission* and *residual state* will be difficult to make.

In Full Remission: There are no longer any symptoms or signs of the disorder. The differentiation of *in full remission* from recovered (no current mental disorder) requires consideration of the length of time since the last period of disturbance, the total duration of the disturbance, and the need for continued evaluation or prophylactic treatment.

The Diagnostic Categories

Disorders Usually First Evident in Infancy, Childhood, or Adolescence

This section lists conditions that are usually first evident in infancy, childhood, or adolescence. However, any adult diagnosis may be used, when appropriate, for diagnosing a child.

DEVELOPMENTAL DISORDERS (Mental Retardation, Pervasive Developmental Disorders, and Specific Developmental Disorders)

Note: These are coded on Axis II.

MENTAL RETARDATION (AXIS II)

A. Significantly subaverage general intellectual functioning: an IQ of 70 or below on an individually administered IQ test (for infants, a clinical judgment of significantly subaverage intellectual functioning, since available intelligence tests do not yield numerical IQ values).

B. Concurrent deficits or impairments in adaptive functioning, i.e., the person's effectiveness in meeting the standards expected for his or her age by his or her cultural group in areas such as social skills and responsibility, communication, daily living skills, personal independence, and self-sufficiency.

C. Onset before the age of 18.

Levels of severity. There are four specific levels of severity, reflecting the degree of intellectual impairment and designated as Mild, Moderate, Severe, and Profound. IQ levels to be used as guides for distinguishing the four levels are given below:

Levels of severity of Mental Retardation	IQ levels
317.00 Mild Mental Retardation	50-55 to approx. 70
318.00 Moderate Mental Retardation	35-40 to 50-55
318.10 Severe Mental Retardation	20-25 to 35-40
318.20 Profound Mental Retardation	Below 20 or 25

319.00 Unspecified Mental Retardation

This category should be used when there is a strong presumption of Mental Retardation, but the person is untestable by standard intelligence tests. This may be the case when children, adolescents, or adults are too impaired or uncooperative to be tested. This may also be the case with infants when there is a clinical judgment of significantly subaverage intellectual functioning, but the available tests, such as the Bayley, Cattel, and others, do not yield IQ values. In general, the younger the age, the more difficult it is to make a diagnosis of Mental Retardation, except for those with profound impairment.

This category should not be used when the intellectual level is presumed to be above 70 (see V code for Borderline Intellectual Functioning, p. 204).

PERVASIVE DEVELOPMENTAL DISORDERS (AXIS II)

299.00 Autistic Disorder

At least eight of the following sixteen items are present, these to include at least two items from A, one from B, and one from C.

Note: Consider a criterion to be met *only* if the behavior is abnormal for the person's developmental level.

A. Qualitative impairment in reciprocal social interaction as manifested by the following:

   (The examples within parentheses are arranged so that those first mentioned are more likely to apply to younger or more handicapped, and the later ones, to older or less handicapped, persons with this disorder.)

   (1) marked lack of awareness of the existence or feelings of others (e.g., treats a person as if he or she were a piece of furniture; does not notice another person's distress; apparently has no concept of the need of others for privacy)

   (2) no or abnormal seeking of comfort at times of distress (e.g., does not come for comfort even when ill, hurt, or tired; seeks comfort in a stereotyped way, e.g., says "cheese, cheese, cheese" whenever hurt)

   (3) no or impaired imitation (e.g., does not wave bye-bye; does not copy mother's domestic activities; mechanical imitation of others' actions out of context)

   (4) no or abnormal social play (e.g., does not actively participate in simple games; prefers solitary play activities; involves other children in play only as "mechanical aids")

(5) gross impairment in ability to make peer friendships (e.g., no interest in making peer friendships; despite interest in making friends, demonstrates lack of understanding of conventions of social interaction, for example, reads phone book to uninterested peer)

B. Qualitative impairment in verbal and nonverbal communication, and in imaginative activity, as manifested by the following:

(The numbered items are arranged so that those first listed are more likely to apply to younger or more handicapped, and the later ones, to older or less handicapped, persons with this disorder.)

(1) no mode of communication, such as communicative babbling, facial expression, gesture, mime, or spoken language

(2) markedly abnormal nonverbal communication, as in the use of eye-to-eye gaze, facial expression, body posture, or gestures to initiate or modulate social interaction (e.g., does not anticipate being held, stiffens when held, does not look at the person or smile when making a social approach, does not greet parents or visitors, has a fixed stare in social situations)

(3) absence of imaginative activity, such as playacting of adult roles, fantasy characters, or animals; lack of interest in stories about imaginary events

(4) marked abnormalities in the production of speech, including volume, pitch, stress, rate, rhythm, and intonation (e.g., monotonous tone, questionlike melody, or high pitch)

(5) marked abnormalities in the form or content of speech, including stereotyped and repetitive use of speech (e.g., immediate echolalia or mechanical repetition of television

commercial); use of "you" when "I" is meant (e.g., using "You want cookie?" to mean "I want a cookie"); idiosyncratic use of words or phrases (e.g., "Go on green riding" to mean "I want to go on the swing"); or frequent irrelevant remarks (e.g., starts talking about train schedules during a conversation about sports)

(6) marked impairment in the ability to initiate or sustain a conversation with others, despite adequate speech (e.g., indulging in lengthy monologues on one subject regardless of interjections from others)

C. Markedly restricted repertoire of activities and interests, as manifested by the following:

(1) stereotyped body movements, e.g., hand-flicking or -twisting, spinning, head-banging, complex whole-body movements

(2) persistent preoccupation with parts of objects (e.g., sniffing or smelling objects, repetitive feeling of texture of materials, spinning wheels of toy cars) or attachment to unusual objects (e.g., insists on carrying around a piece of string)

(3) marked distress over changes in trivial aspects of environment, e.g., when a vase is moved from usual position

(4) unreasonable insistence on following routines in precise detail, e.g., insisting that exactly the same route always be followed when shopping

(5) markedly restricted range of interests and a preoccupation with one narrow interest, e.g., interested only in lining up objects, in amassing facts about meteorology, or in pretending to be a fantasy character

D. Onset during infancy or childhood.

Specify if childhood onset (after 36 months of age).

299.80 Pervasive Developmental Disorder Not Otherwise Specified

This category should be used when there is a qualitative impairment in the development of reciprocal social interaction and of verbal and nonverbal communication skills, but the criteria are not met for Autistic Disorder, Schizophrenia, or Schizotypal or Schizoid Personality Disorder. Some people with this diagnosis will exhibit a markedly restricted repertoire of activities and interests, but others will not.

SPECIFIC DEVELOPMENTAL DISORDERS (AXIS II)

Academic Skills Disorders

315.10 Developmental Arithmetic Disorder

A. Arithmetic skills, as measured by a standardized, individually administered test, are markedly below the expected level, given the person's schooling and intellectual capacity (as determined by an individually administered IQ test).

B. The disturbance in A significantly interferes with academic achievement or activities of daily living requiring arithmetic skills.

C. Not due to a defect in visual or hearing acuity or a neurologic disorder.

315.80 Developmental Expressive Writing Disorder

A. Writing skills, as measured by a standardized, individually administered test, are markedly below the expected level, given the person's schooling and intellectual capacity (as determined by an individually administered IQ test).

B. The disturbance in A significantly interferes with academic achievement or activities of daily living requiring the composition of written texts (spelling words and expressing thoughts in grammatically correct sentences and organized paragraphs).

C. Not due to a defect in visual or hearing acuity or a neurologic disorder.

315.00 Developmental Reading Disorder

A. Reading achievement, as measured by a standardized, individually administered test, is markedly below the expected level, given the person's schooling and intellectual capacity (as determined by an individually administered IQ test).

B. The disturbance in A significantly interferes with academic achievement or activities of daily living requiring reading skills.

C. Not due to a defect in visual or hearing acuity or a neurologic disorder.

Language and Speech Disorders

315.39 Developmental Articulation Disorder

A. Consistent failure to use developmentally expected speech sounds. For example, in a three-year-old, failure to articulate p, b, and t, and in a six-year-old, failure to articulate r, sh, th, f, z, and l.

B. Not due to a Pervasive Developmental Disorder, Mental Retardation, defect in hearing acuity, disorders of the oral speech mechanism, or a neurologic disorder.

315.31 Developmental Expressive Language Disorder

A. The score obtained from a standardized measure of expressive language is substantially below that obtained from a standardized measure of nonverbal intellectual capacity (as determined by an individually administered IQ test).

B. The disturbance in A significantly interferes with academic achievement or activities of daily living requiring the expression of verbal (or sign) language. This may be evidenced in severe cases by use of a markedly limited vocabulary, by speaking only in simple sentences, or by speaking only in the present tense. In less severe cases, there may be hesitations or errors in recalling certain words, or errors in the production of long or complex sentences.

C. Not due to a Pervasive Developmental Disorder, defect in hearing acuity, or a neurologic disorder (aphasia).

315.31 Developmental Receptive Language Disorder

A. The score obtained from a standardized measure of receptive language is substantially below that obtained from a standardized measure of nonverbal intellectual capacity (as determined by an individually administered IQ test).

B. The disturbance in A significantly interferes with academic achievement or activities of daily living requiring the comprehension of verbal (or sign) language. This may be manifested in more severe cases by an inability to understand simple words or sentences. In less severe cases, there may be difficulty in understanding only certain types of words, such as spatial terms, or an inability to comprehend longer or more complex statements.

C. Not due to a Pervasive Developmental Disorder, defect in hearing acuity, or a neurologic disorder (aphasia).

Motor Skills Disorder

315.40 Developmental Coordination Disorder

A. The person's performance in daily activities requiring motor coordination is markedly below the expected level, given the person's chronological age and intellectual capacity. This may be manifested by marked delays in achieving motor milestones (walking, crawling, sitting), dropping things, "clumsiness," poor performance in sports, or poor handwriting.

B. The disturbance in A significantly interferes with academic achievement or activities of daily living.

C. Not due to a known physical disorder, such as cerebral palsy, hemiplegia, or muscular dystrophy.

315.90 Specific Developmental Disorder Not Otherwise Specified

Disorders in the development of language, speech, academic, and motor skills that do not meet the criteria for a Specific Developmental Disorder. Examples include aphasia with epilepsy acquired in childhood ("Landau syndrome") and specific developmental difficulties in spelling.

OTHER DEVELOPMENTAL DISORDERS (AXIS II)

315.90 Developmental Disorder Not Otherwise Specified

Disorders in development that do not meet the criteria for either Mental Retardation or a Pervasive or a Specific Developmental Disorder.

DISRUPTIVE BEHAVIOR DISORDERS

314.01 Attention-deficit Hyperactivity Disorder

Note: Consider a criterion met only if the behavior is considerably more frequent than that of most people of the same mental age.

A. A disturbance of at least six months during which at least eight of the following are present:

    (1) often fidgets with hands or feet or squirms in seat (in adolescents, may be limited to subjective feelings of restlessness)

    (2) has difficulty remaining seated when required to do so

    (3) is easily distracted by extraneous stimuli

    (4) has difficulty awaiting turn in games or group situations

    (5) often blurts out answers to questions before they have been completed

    (6) has difficulty following through on instructions from others (not due to oppositional behavior or failure of comprehension), e.g., fails to finish chores

    (7) has difficulty sustaining attention in tasks or play activities

    (8) often shifts from one uncompleted activity to another

(9) has difficulty playing quietly

(10) often talks excessively

(11) often interrupts or intrudes on others, e.g., butts into other children's games

(12) often does not seem to listen to what is being said to him or her

(13) often loses things necessary for tasks or activities at school or at home (e.g., toys, pencils, books, assignments)

(14) often engages in physically dangerous activities without considering possible consequences (not for the purpose of thrill-seeking), e.g., runs into street without looking

Note: The above items are listed in descending order of discriminating power based on data from a national field trial of the DSM-III-R criteria for Disruptive Behavior Disorders.

B. Onset before the age of seven.

C. Does not meet the criteria for a Pervasive Developmental Disorder.

Criteria for severity of Attention-deficit Hyperactivity Disorder:

Mild: Few, if any, symptoms in excess of those required to make the diagnosis **and** only minimal or no impairment in school and social functioning.

Moderate: Symptoms or functional impairment intermediate between "mild" and "severe."

Severe: Many symptoms in excess of those required to make the diagnosis **and** significant and pervasive impairment in functioning at home and school and with peers.

Conduct Disorder

A. A disturbance of conduct lasting at least six months, during which at least three of the following have been present:

   (1) has stolen without confrontation of a victim on more than one occasion (including forgery)

   (2) has run away from home overnight at least twice while living in parental or parental surrogate home (or once without returning)

   (3) often lies (other than to avoid physical or sexual abuse)

   (4) has deliberately engaged in fire-setting

   (5) is often truant from school (for older person, absent from work)

   (6) has broken into someone else's house, building, or car

   (7) has deliberately destroyed others' property (other than by fire-setting)

   (8) has been physically cruel to animals

   (9) has forced someone into sexual activity with him or her

  (10) has used a weapon in more than one fight

  (11) often initiates physical fights

  (12) has stolen with confrontation of a victim (e.g., mugging, purse-snatching, extortion, armed robbery)

  (13) has been physically cruel to people

Note: The above items are listed in descending order of discriminating power based on data from a national field trial of the DSM-III-R criteria for Disruptive Behavior Disorders.

B. If 18 or older, does not meet criteria for Antisocial Personality Disorder.

Criteria for severity of Conduct Disorder:

Mild: Few if any conduct problems in excess of those required to make the diagnosis, **and** conduct problems cause only minor harm to others.

Moderate: Number of conduct problems and effect on others intermediate between "mild" and "severe."

Severe: Many conduct problems in excess of those required to make the diagnosis, **or** conduct problems cause considerable harm to others, e.g., serious physical injury to victims, extensive vandalism or theft, prolonged absence from home.

Types

312.20 group type

The essential feature is the predominance of conduct problems occurring mainly as a group activity with peers. Aggressive physical behavior may or may not be present.

312.00 solitary aggressive type

The essential feature is the predominance of aggressive physical behavior, usually toward both adults and peers, initiated by the person (not as a group activity).

312.90 undifferentiated type

This a subtype for children or adolescents with Conduct Disorder with a mixture of clinical features that cannot be classified as either Solitary Aggressive Type or Group Type.

313.81 Oppositional Defiant Disorder

Note: Consider a criterion met only if the behavior is considerably more frequent than that of most people of the same mental age.

A. A disturbance of at least six months during which at least five of the following are present:

    (1) often loses temper

    (2) often argues with adults

    (3) often actively defies or refuses adult requests or rules, e.g., refuses to do chores at home

    (4) often deliberately does things that annoy other people, e.g., grabs other children's hats

    (5) often blames others for his or her own mistakes

    (6) is often touchy or easily annoyed by others

    (7) is often angry and resentful

    (8) is often spiteful or vindictive

    (9) often swears or uses obscene language

Note: The above items are listed in descending order of discriminating power based on data from a national field trial of the DSM-III-R criteria for Disruptive Behavior Disorders.

B. Does not meet the criteria for Conduct Disorder, and does not occur exclusively during the course of a psychotic disorder, Dysthymia, or a Major Depressive, Hypomanic, or Manic Episode.

Criteria for severity of Oppositional Defiant Disorder:

Mild: Few, if any, symptoms in excess of those required to make the diagnosis **and** only minimal or no impairment in school and social functioning.

Moderate: Symptoms or functional impairment intermediate between "mild" and "severe."

Severe: Many symptoms in excess of those required to make the diagnosis **and** significant and pervasive impairment in functioning at home and school and with other adults and peers.

ANXIETY DISORDERS OF CHILDHOOD OR ADOLESCENCE

309.21 Separation Anxiety Disorder

A. Excessive anxiety concerning separation from those to whom the child is attached, as evidenced by at least three of the following:

   (1) unrealistic and persistent worry about possible harm befalling major attachment figures or fear that they will leave and not return

   (2) unrealistic and persistent worry that an untoward calamitous event will separate the child from a major attachment figure, e.g., the child will be lost, kidnapped, killed, or be the victim of an accident

   (3) persistent reluctance or refusal to go to school in order to stay with major attachment figures or at home

   (4) persistent reluctance or refusal to go to sleep without being near a major attachment figure or to go to sleep away from home

   (5) persistent avoidance of being alone, including "clinging" to and "shadowing" major attachment figures

   (6) repeated nightmares involving the theme of separation

   (7) complaints of physical symptoms, e.g., headaches, stomachaches, nausea, or vomiting, on many school days or on other occasions when anticipating separation from major attachment figures

   (8) recurrent signs or complaints of excessive distress in anticipation of separation from home

or major attachment figures, e.g., temper tantrums or crying, pleading with parents not to leave

(9) recurrent signs of complaints of excessive distress when separated from home or major attachment figures, e.g., wants to return home, needs to call parents when they are absent or when child is away from home

B. Duration of disturbance of at least two weeks.

C. Onset before the age of 18.

D. Occurrence not exclusively during the course of a Pervasive Developmental Disorder, Schizophrenia, or any other psychotic disorder.

313.21 Avoidant Disorder of Childhood or Adolescence

A. Excessive shrinking from contact with unfamiliar people, for a period of six months or longer, sufficiently severe to interfere with social functioning in peer relationships.

B. Desire for social involvement with familiar people (family members and peers the person knows well), and generally warm and satisfying relations with family members and other familiar figures.

C. Age at least 2½ years.

D. The disturbance is not sufficiently pervasive and persistent to warrant the diagnosis of Avoidant Personality Disorder.

313.00 Overanxious Disorder

A. Excessive or unrealistic anxiety or worry, for a period of six months or longer, as indicated by the frequent occurrence of at least four of the following:

   (1) excessive or unrealistic worry about future events

   (2) excessive or unrealistic concern about the appropriateness of past behavior

   (3) excessive or unrealistic concern about competence in one or more areas, e.g., athletic, academic, social

   (4) somatic complaints, such as headaches or stomachaches, for which no physical basis can be established

   (5) marked self-consciousness

   (6) excessive need for reassurance about a variety of concerns

   (7) marked feelings of tension or inability to relax

B. If another Axis I disorder is present (e.g., Separation Anxiety Disorder, Phobic Disorder, Obsessive Compulsive Disorder), the focus of the symptoms in A are not limited to it. For example, if Separation Anxiety Disorder is present, the symptoms in A are not exclusively related to anxiety about separation. In addition, the disturbance does not occur only during the course of a psychotic disorder or a Mood Disorder.

C. If 18 or older, does not meet the criteria for Generalized Anxiety Disorder.

D. Occurrence not exclusively during the course of a Pervasive Developmental Disorder, Schizophrenia, or any other psychotic disorder.

EATING DISORDERS

307.10 Anorexia Nervosa

A. Refusal to maintain body weight over a minimal normal weight for age and height, e.g., weight loss leading to maintenance of body weight 15% below that expected; or failure to make expected weight gain during period of growth, leading to body weight 15% below that expected.

B. Intense fear of gaining weight or becoming fat, even though underweight.

C. Disturbance in the way in which one's body weight, size, or shape is experienced, e.g., the person claims to "feel fat" even when emaciated, believes that one area of the body is "too fat" even when obviously underweight.

D. In females, absence of at least three consecutive menstrual cycles when otherwise expected to occur (primary or secondary amenorrhea). (A woman is considered to have amenorrhea if her periods occur only following hormone, e.g., estrogen, administration.)

307.51 Bulimia Nervosa

A. Recurrent episodes of binge eating (rapid consumption of a large amount of food in a discrete period of time).

B. A feeling of lack of control over eating behavior during the eating binges.

C. The person regularly engages in either self-induced vomiting, use of laxatives or diuretics, strict dieting or fasting, or vigorous exercise in order to prevent weight gain.

D. A minimum average of two binge eating episodes a week for at least three months.

E. Persistent overconcern with body shape and weight.

307.52 Pica

A. Repeated eating of a nonnutritive substance for at least one month.

B. Does not meet the criteria for either Autistic Disorder, Schizophrenia, or Kleine-Levin syndrome.

307.53 Rumination Disorder of Infancy

A. Repeated regurgitation, without nausea or associated gastrointestinal illness, for at least one month following a period of normal functioning.

B. Weight loss or failure to make expected weight gain.

307.50 Eating Disorder Not Otherwise Specified

Disorders of eating that do not meet the criteria for a specific Eating Disorder.

Examples:

(1) a person of average weight who does not have binge eating episodes, but frequently engages in self-induced vomiting for fear of gaining weight
(2) all of the features of Anorexia Nervosa in a female except absence of menses
(3) all of the features of Bulimia Nervosa except the frequency of binge eating episodes

GENDER IDENTITY DISORDERS

302.60 Gender Identity Disorder of Childhood

For Females:

A. Persistent and intense distress about being a girl, and a stated desire to be a boy (not merely a desire for any perceived cultural advantages from being a boy), or insistence that she is a boy.

B. Either (1) or (2):

(1) persistent marked aversion to normative feminine clothing and insistence on wearing stereotypical masculine clothing, e.g., boys' underwear and other accessories

(2) persistent repudiation of female anatomic structures, as evidenced by at least one of the following:

(a) an assertion that she has, or will grow, a penis

(b) rejection of urinating in a sitting position

(c) assertion that she does not want to grow breasts or menstruate

C. The girl has not yet reached puberty.

For Males:

A. Persistent and intense distress about being a boy and an intense desire to be a girl or, more rarely, insistence that he is a girl.

B. Either (1) or (2):

(1) preoccupation with female stereotypical activities, as shown by a preference for either cross-dressing or simulating female attire, or by an intense desire to participate in the games and pastimes of girls and rejection of male stereotypical toys, games, and activities

(2) persistent repudiation of male anatomic structures, as indicated by at least one of the following repeated assertions:

(a) that he will grow up to become a woman (not merely in role)

(b) that his penis or testes are disgusting or will disappear

(c) that it would be better not to have a penis or testes

C. The boy has not yet reached puberty.

302.50 Transsexualism

A. Persistent discomfort and sense of inappropriateness about one's assigned sex.

B. Persistent preoccupation for at least two years with getting rid of one's primary and secondary sex characteristics and acquiring the sex characteristics of the other sex.

C. The person has reached puberty.

Specify history of sexual orientation: **asexual, homosexual, heterosexual,** or **unspecified.**

302.85 Gender Identity Disorder of Adolescence or Adulthood, Nontranssexual Type (GIDAANT)

A. Persistent or recurrent discomfort and sense of inappropriateness about one's assigned sex.

B. Persistent or recurrent cross-dressing in the role of the other sex, either in fantasy or actuality, but not for the purpose of sexual excitement (as in Transvestic Fetishism).

C. No persistent preoccupation (for at least two years) with getting rid of one's primary and secondary sex characteristics and acquiring the sex characteristics of the other sex (as in Transsexualism).

D. The person has reached puberty.

Specify history of sexual orientation: **asexual, homosexual, heterosexual,** or **unspecified.**

302.85 Gender Identity Disorder Not Otherwise Specified

Disorders in gender identity that are not classifiable as a specific Gender Identity Disorder.

Examples:

(1) children with persistent cross-dressing without the other criteria for Gender Identity Disorder of Childhood
(2) adults with transient, stress-related cross-dressing behavior
(3) adults with the clinical features of Transsexualism of less than two years' duration
(4) people who have a persistent preoccupation with castration or peotomy without a desire to acquire the sex characteristics of the other sex

TIC DISORDERS

A tic is an involuntary, sudden, rapid, recurrent, non-rhythmic, stereotyped, motor movement or vocalization. It is experienced as irresistible, but can be suppressed for varying lengths of time. All forms of tics are often exacerbated by stress and usually are markedly diminished during sleep. They may become attenuated during some absorbing activities, such as reading or sewing.

Both *motor* and *vocal* tics may be classified as either *simple* or *complex*, although the boundaries are not well defined. Common *simple motor tics* are eye-blinking, neck-jerking, shoulder-shrugging, and facial grimacing. Common *simple vocal tics* are coughing, throat-clearing, grunting, sniffing, snorting, and barking. Common *complex motor tics* are facial gestures, grooming behaviors, hitting or biting self, jumping, touching, stamping, and smelling an object. Common *complex vocal tics* are repeating words or phrases out of context, coprolalia (use of socially unacceptable words, frequently obscene), palilalia (repeating one's own sounds or words), and echolalia (repeating the last-heard sound, word, or phrase of another person, or last-heard sound). Other complex tics include echokinesis (imitation of the movements of someone who is being observed).

307.23 Tourette's Disorder

A. Both multiple motor and one or more vocal tics have been present at some time during the illness, although not necessarily concurrently.

B. The tics occur many times a day (usually in bouts), nearly every day or intermittently throughout a period of more than one year.

C. The anatomic location, number, frequency, complexity, and severity of the tics change over time.

D. Onset before age 21.

E. Occurrence not exclusively during Psychoactive Substance Intoxication or known central nervous system disease, such as Huntington's chorea and postviral encephalitis.

307.22 Chronic Motor or Vocal Tic Disorder

A. Either motor or vocal tics, but not both, have been present at some time during the illness.

B. The tics occur many times a day, nearly every day, or intermittently throughout a period of more than one year.

C. Onset before age 21.

D. Occurrence not exclusively during Psychoactive Substance Intoxication or known central nervous system disease, such as Huntington's chorea and postviral encephalitis.

307.21 Transient Tic Disorder

A. Single or multiple motor and/or vocal tics.

B. The tics occur many times a day, nearly every day for at least two weeks, but for no longer than twelve consecutive months.

C. No history of Tourette's or Chronic Motor or Vocal Tic Disorder.

D. Onset before age 21.

E. Occurrence not exclusively during Psychoactive Substance Intoxication or known central nervous system disease, such as Huntington's chorea and postviral encephalitis.

Specify: single episode or **recurrent.**

307.20 Tic Disorder Not Otherwise Specified

Tics that do not meet the criteria for a specific Tic Disorder. An example is a Tic Disorder with onset in adulthood.

ELIMINATION DISORDERS

307.70 Functional Encopresis

A. Repeated passage of feces into places not appropriate for that purpose (e.g., clothing, floor), whether involuntary or intentional. (The disorder may be overflow incontinence secondary to functional fecal retention.)

B. At least one such event a month for at least six months.

C. Chronologic and mental age, at least four years.

D. Not due to a physical disorder, such as aganglionic megacolon.

Specify primary or secondary type.

Primary type: the disturbance was not preceded by a period of fecal continence lasting at least one year.

Secondary type: the disturbance was preceded by a period of fecal continence lasting at least one year.

307.60 Functional Enuresis

A. Repeated voiding of urine during the day or night into bed or clothes, whether involuntary or intentional.

B. At least two such events per month for children between the ages of five and six, and at least one event per month for older children.

C. Chronologic age at least five, and mental age at least four.

D. Not due to a physical disorder, such as diabetes, urinary tract infection, or a seizure disorder.

Specify primary or secondary type.

Primary type: the disturbance was not preceded by a period of urinary continence lasting at least one year.

Secondary type: the disturbance was preceded by a period of urinary continence lasting at least one year.

Specify nocturnal only, diurnal only, or **nocturnal and diurnal.**

SPEECH DISORDERS NOT ELSEWHERE CLASSIFIED

307.00 Cluttering

A disorder of speech fluency involving both the rate and the rhythm of speech and resulting in impaired speech intelligibility. Speech is erratic and dysrhythmic, consisting of rapid and jerky spurts that usually involve faulty phrasing patterns (e.g., alternating pauses and bursts of speech that produce groups of words unrelated to the grammatical structure of the sentence).

307.00 Stuttering

Frequent repetitions or prolongations of sounds or syllables that markedly impair the fluency of speech.

OTHER DISORDERS OF INFANCY, CHILDHOOD, OR ADOLESCENCE

313.23 Elective Mutism

A. Persistent refusal to talk in one or more major social situations (including at school).

B. Ability to comprehend spoken language and to speak.

313.82 Identity Disorder

A. Severe subjective distress regarding uncertainty about a variety of issues relating to identity, including three or more of the following:

    (1) long-term goals

    (2) career choice

    (3) friendship patterns

    (4) sexual orientation and behavior

    (5) religious identification

    (6) moral value systems
    (7) group loyalties

B. Impairment in social or occupational (including academic) functioning as a result of the symptoms in A.

C. Duration of the disturbance of at least three months.

D. Occurrence not exclusively during the course of a Mood Disorder or of a psychotic disorder, such as Schizophrenia.

E The disturbance is not sufficiently pervasive and persistent to warrant the diagnosis of Borderline Personality Disorder.

313.89 Reactive Attachment Disorder of Infancy or Early Childhood

A. Markedly disturbed social relatedness in most contexts, beginning before the age of five, as evidenced by either (1) or (2):

    (1) persistent failure to initiate or respond to most social interactions (e.g., in infants, absence of visual tracking and reciprocal play, lack of vocal imitation or playfulness, apathy, little or no spontaneity; at later ages, lack of or little curiosity and social interest)

    (2) indiscriminate sociability, e.g., excessive familiarity with relative strangers by making requests and displaying affection

B. The disturbance in A is not a symptom of either Mental Retardation or a Pervasive Developmental Disorder, such as Autistic Disorder.

C. Grossly pathogenic care, as evidenced by at least one of the following:

  (1) persistent disregard of the child's basic emotional needs for comfort, stimulation, and affection. *Examples*: overly harsh punishment by caregiver; consistent neglect by caregiver.
  (2) persistent disregard of the child's basic physical needs, including nutrition, adequate housing, and protection from physical danger and assault (including sexual abuse)
  (3) repeated change of primary caregiver so that stable attachments are not possible, e.g., frequent changes in foster parents

D. There is a presumption that the care described in C is responsible for the disturbed behavior in A; this presumption is warranted if the disturbance in A began following the pathogenic care in C.

Note: If failure to thrive is present, code it on Axis III.

307.30 Stereotypy/Habit Disorder

A. Intentional, repetitive, nonfunctional behaviors, such as hand-shaking or -waving, body-rocking, head-banging, mouthing of objects, nail-biting, picking at nose or skin.

B. The disturbance either causes physical injury to the child or markedly interferes with normal activities, e.g., injury to head from head-banging; inability to fall asleep because of constant rocking.

C. Does not meet the criteria for either a Pervasive Developmental Disorder or a Tic Disorder.

314.00 Undifferentiated Attention-deficit Disorder

This is a residual category for disturbances in which the predominant feature is the persistence of developmentally inappropriate and marked inattention that is not a symptom of another disorder, such as Mental Retardation or Attention-deficit Hyperactivity Disorder, or of a disorganized and chaotic environment. Some of the disturbances that in DSM-III would have been categorized as Attention-deficit Disorder without Hyperactivity would be included in this category. Research is necessary to determine if this is a valid diagnostic category and, if so, how it should be defined.

Organic Mental Syndromes and Disorders

In the following section, criteria are provided for the various Organic Mental Syndromes. These are followed by criteria for the specific Organic Mental Disorders.

ORGANIC MENTAL SYNDROMES

Delirium

A. Reduced ability to maintain attention to external stimuli (e.g., questions must be repeated because attention wanders) and to appropriately shift attention to new external stimuli (e.g., perseverates answer to a previous question).

B. Disorganized thinking, as indicated by rambling, irrelevant, or incoherent speech.

C. At least two of the following:

    (1) reduced level of consciousness, e.g., difficulty keeping awake during examination
    (2) perceptual disturbances: misinterpretations, illusions, or hallucinations
    (3) disturbance of sleep-wake cycle with insomnia or daytime sleepiness
    (4) increased or decreased psychomotor activity
    (5) disorientation to time, place, or person

    (6) memory impairment, e.g., inability to learn new material, such as the names of several unrelated objects, after five minutes, or to remember past events, such as history of current episode of illness

D. Clinical features develop over a short period of time (usually hours to days) and tend to fluctuate over the course of a day.

E. Either (1) or (2):

    (1) evidence from the history, physical examination, or laboratory tests of a specific organic factor (or factors) judged to be etiologically related to the disturbance

    (2) in the absence of such evidence, an etiologic organic factor can be presumed if the disturbance cannot be accounted for by any non-organic mental disorder, e.g., Manic Episode accounting for agitation and sleep disturbance

Dementia

A. Demonstrable evidence of impairment in short- and long-term memory. Impairment in short-term memory (inability to learn new information) may be indicated by inability to remember three objects after five minutes. Long-term memory impairment (inability to remember information that was known in the past) may be indicated by inability to remember past personal information (e.g., what happened yesterday, birthplace, occupation) or facts of common knowledge (e.g., past Presidents, well-known dates).

B. At least one of the following:

    (1) impairment in abstract thinking, as indicated by inability to find similarities and differences

between related words, difficulty in defining words and concepts, and other similar tasks

(2) impaired judgment, as indicated by inability to make reasonable plans to deal with interpersonal, family, and job-related problems and issues

(3) other disturbances of higher cortical function, such as aphasia (disorder of language), apraxia (inability to carry out motor activities despite intact comprehension and motor function), agnosia (failure to recognize or identify objects despite intact sensory function), and "constructional difficulty" (e.g., inability to copy three-dimensional figures, assemble blocks, or arrange sticks in specific designs)

(4) personality change, i.e., alteration or accentuation of premorbid traits

C. The disturbance in A and B significantly interferes with work or usual social activities or relationships with others.

D. Not occurring exclusively during the course of Delirium.

E. Either (1) or (2):

(1) there is evidence from the history, physical examination, or laboratory tests of a specific organic factor (or factors) judged to be etiologically related to the disturbance

(2) in the absence of such evidence, an etiologic organic factor can be presumed if the disturbance cannot be accounted for by any non-organic mental disorder, e.g., Major Depression accounting for cognitive impairment

Criteria for severity of Dementia:

Mild: Although work or social activities are significantly impaired, the capacity for independent living remains, with adequate personal hygiene and relatively intact judgment.

Moderate: Independent living is hazardous, and some degree of supervision is necessary.

Severe: Activities of daily living are so impaired that continual supervision is required, e.g., unable to maintain minimal personal hygiene; largely incoherent or mute.

Amnestic Syndrome

A. Demonstrable evidence of impairment in both short- and long-term memory; with regard to long-term memory, very remote events are remembered better than more recent events. Impairment in short-term memory (inability to learn new information) may be indicated by inability to remember three objects after five minutes. Long-term memory impairment (inability to remember information that was known in the past) may be indicated by inability to remember past personal information (e.g., what happened yesterday, birthplace, occupation) or facts of common knowledge (e.g., past Presidents, well-known dates).

B. Not occurring exclusively during the course of Delirium, and does not meet the criteria for Dementia (i.e., no impairment in abstract thinking or judgment, no other disturbances of higher cortical function, and no personality change).

C. There is evidence from the history, physical examination, or laboratory tests of a specific organic

factor (or factors) judged to be etiologically related
to the disturbance.

Organic Delusional Syndrome

A. Prominent delusions.

B. There is evidence from the history, physical examination, or laboratory tests of a specific organic
factor (or factors) judged to be etiologically related
to the disturbance.

C. Not occurring exclusively during the course of
Delirium.

Organic Hallucinosis

A. Prominent persistent or recurrent hallucinations.

B. There is evidence from the history, physical examination, or laboratory tests of a specific organic
factor (or factors) judged to be etiologically related
to the disturbance.

C. Not occurring exclusively during the course of
Delirium.

Organic Mood Syndrome

A. Prominent and persistent depressed, elevated, or
expansive mood.

B. There is evidence from the history, physical examination, or laboratory tests of a specific organic
factor (or factors) judged to be etiologically related
to the disturbance.

C. Not occurring exclusively during the course of
Delirium.

Specify: manic, depressed, or **mixed.**

Organic Anxiety Syndrome

A. Prominent, recurrent, panic attacks (criteria A, C, and D of Panic Disorder, p. 139) or generalized anxiety (criterion D of Generalized Anxiety Disorder, p. 148).

B. There is evidence from the history, physical examination, or laboratory tests of a specific organic factor (or factors) judged to be etiologically related to the disturbance.

C. Not occurring exclusively during the course of Delirium.

Organic Personality Syndrome

A. A persistent personality disturbance, either life-long or representing a change or accentuation of a previously characteristic trait, involving at least one of the following:

(1) affective instability, e.g., marked shifts from normal mood to depression, irritability, or anxiety

(2) recurrent outbursts of aggression or rage that are grossly out of proportion to any precipitating psychosocial stressors

(3) markedly impaired social judgment, e.g., sexual indiscretions

(4) marked apathy and indifference

(5) suspiciousness or paranoid ideation

B. There is evidence from the history, physical examination, or laboratory tests of a specific organic factor (or factors) judged to be etiologically related to the disturbance.

C. This diagnosis is not given to a child or adolescent if the clinical picture is limited to the features that characterize Attention-deficit Hyperactivity Disorder (see p. 56).

D. Not occurring exclusively during the course of Delirium, and does not meet the criteria for Dementia.

Specify explosive type if outbursts of aggression or rage are the predominant feature.

Intoxication

A. Development of a substance-specific syndrome due to recent ingestion of a psychoactive substance. (**Note:** More than one substance may produce similar or identical syndromes.)

B. Maladaptive behavior during the waking state due to the effect of the substance on the central nervous system, e.g., belligerence, impaired judgment, impaired social or occupational functioning.

C. The clinical picture does not correspond to any of the other specific Organic Mental Syndromes, such as Delirium, Organic Delusional Syndrome, Organic Hallucinosis, Organic Mood Syndrome, or Organic Anxiety Syndrome.

Withdrawal

A. Development of a substance-specific syndrome that follows the cessation of, or reduction in, intake of a psychoactive substance that the person previously used regularly.

B. The clinical picture does not correspond to any of the other specific Organic Mental Syndromes, such as Delirium, Organic Delusional Syndrome, Organic Hallucinosis, Organic Mood Syndrome, or Organic Anxiety Syndrome.

Organic Mental Syndrome Not Otherwise Specified

Organic Mental Syndromes that do not meet the criteria for any of the previously described categories.

Examples:

(1) "neurasthenic" picture associated with early Addison's disease
(2) unusual disturbances of consciousness or behavior occurring during seizures

ORGANIC MENTAL DISORDERS

DEMENTIAS ARISING IN THE SENIUM AND PRESENIUM

Primary Degenerative Dementia of the Alzheimer Type

Note: Code 331.00 Alzheimer's Disease on Axis III.

A. Dementia (see p. 78).

B. Insidious onset with a generally progressive deteriorating course.

C. Exclusion of all other specific causes of Dementia by history, physical examination, and laboratory tests.

Types

Primary Degenerative Dementia of the Alzheimer Type, Senile Onset (after age 65)

290.30 with delirium

290.20 with delusions

290.21 with depression

290.00 uncomplicated

Primary Degenerative Dementia of the Alzheimer Type, Presenile Onset (age 65 and below)

290.11 with delirium

290.12 with delusions

290.13 with depression

290.10 uncomplicated

Multi-infarct Dementia

A. Dementia (see p. 78).

B. Stepwise deteriorating course with "patchy" distribution of deficits (i.e., affecting some functions, but not others) early in the course.

C. Focal neurologic signs and symptoms (e.g., exaggeration of deep tendon reflexes, extensor plantar response, pseudobulbar palsy, gait abnormalities, weakness of an extremity, etc.).

D. Evidence from history, physical examination, or laboratory tests of significant cerebrovascular disease (recorded on Axis III) that is judged to be etiologically related to the disturbance.

Types

Multi-infarct Dementia

290.41 with delirium

290.42 with delusions

290.43 with depression

290.40 uncomplicated

290.00 Senile Dementia Not Otherwise Specified

Note: Specify etiology on Axis III if known.

Dementias associated with an organic factor and arising after age 65 that cannot be classified as a specific Dementia, e.g., as Primary Degenerative Dementia of the Alzheimer Type, Senile Onset, or Dementia Associated with Alcoholism.

290.10 Presenile Dementia Not Otherwise Specified

Note: Specify etiology on Axis III if known (e.g., Pick's disease, Jakob-Creutzfeldt disease).

Dementias associated with an organic factor and arising before age 65 that cannot be classified as a specific Dementia, e.g., Primary Degenerative Dementia of the Alzheimer Type, Presenile Onset.

PSYCHOACTIVE SUBSTANCE-INDUCED ORGANIC MENTAL DISORDERS

ALCOHOL-INDUCED ORGANIC MENTAL DISORDERS

303.00 Alcohol Intoxication

A. Recent ingestion of alcohol (with no evidence suggesting that the amount was insufficient to cause intoxication in most people).

B. Maladaptive behavioral changes, e.g., disinhibition of sexual or aggressive impulses, mood lability, impaired judgment, impaired social or occupational functioning.

C. At least one of the following signs:

    (1) slurred speech
    (2) incoordination
    (3) unsteady gait
    (4) nystagmus
    (5) flushed face

D. Not due to any physical or other mental disorder.

291.40 Alcohol Idiosyncratic Intoxication

A. Maladaptive behavioral changes, e.g., aggressive or assaultive behavior, occurring within minutes of ingesting an amount of alcohol insufficient to induce intoxication in most people.

B. The behavior is atypical of the person when not drinking.

C. Not due to any physical or other mental disorder.

291.80 Uncomplicated Alcohol Withdrawal

A. Cessation of prolonged (several days or longer) heavy ingestion of alcohol or reduction in the amount of alcohol ingested, followed within several hours by coarse tremor of hands, tongue, or eyelids, and at least one of the following:

    (1) nausea or vomiting
    (2) malaise or weakness
    (3) autonomic hyperactivity, e.g., tachycardia, sweating, elevated blood pressure
    (4) anxiety
    (5) depressed mood or irritability
    (6) transient hallucinations or illusions

(7) headache

(8) insomnia

B. Not due to any physical or other mental disorder, such as Alcohol Withdrawal Delirium.

291.00 Alcohol Withdrawal Delirium

A. Delirium (p. 77) developing after cessation of heavy alcohol ingestion or a reduction in the amount of alcohol ingested (usually within one week).

B. Marked autonomic hyperactivity, e.g., tachycardia, sweating.

C. Not due to any physical or other mental disorder.

291.30 Alcohol Hallucinosis

A. Organic Hallucinosis (p. 81) with vivid and persistent hallucinations (auditory or visual) developing shortly (usually within 48 hours) after cessation of or reduction in heavy ingestion of alcohol in a person who apparently has Alcohol Dependence.

B. No Delirium as in Alcohol Withdrawal Delirium.

C. Not due to any physical or other mental disorder.

291.10 Alcohol Amnestic Disorder

A. Amnestic Syndrome (p. 80) following prolonged, heavy ingestion of alcohol.

B. Not due to any physical or other mental disorder.

291.20 Dementia Associated with Alcoholism

A. Dementia (p. 78) following prolonged, heavy ingestion of alcohol and persisting at least three weeks after cessation of alcohol ingestion.

B. Exclusion by history, physical examination, and laboratory tests, of all causes of Dementia other than prolonged, heavy use of alcohol.

AMPHETAMINE OR SIMILARLY ACTING SYMPATHOMIMETIC-INDUCED ORGANIC MENTAL DISORDERS

305.70 Amphetamine or Similarly Acting Sympathomimetic Intoxication

A. Recent use of amphetamine or a similarly acting sympathomimetic.

B. Maladaptive behavioral changes, e.g., fighting, grandiosity, hypervigilance, psychomotor agitation, impaired judgment, impaired social or occupational functioning.

C. At least two of the following signs within one hour of use:

   (1) tachycardia
   (2) pupillary dilation
   (3) elevated blood pressure
   (4) perspiration or chills
   (5) nausea or vomiting

D. Not due to any physical or other mental disorder.

Note: When the differential diagnosis must be made without a clear-cut history or toxicologic analysis of body fluids, it may be qualified as "Provisional."

292.00 Amphetamine or Similarly Acting Sympathomimetic Withdrawal

A. Cessation of prolonged (several days or longer) heavy use of amphetamine or a similarly acting sympathomimetic, or reduction in the amount of substance used, followed by dysphoric mood (e.g., depression, irritability, anxiety) and at least one of the following, persisting more than 24 hours after cessation of substance use:

(1) fatigue
(2) insomnia or hypersomnia
(3) psychomotor agitation

B. Not due to any physical or other mental disorder, such as Amphetamine or Similarly Acting Sympathomimetic Delusional Disorder.

Note: When the differential diagnosis must be made without a clear-cut history or toxicologic analysis of body fluids, it may be qualified as "Provisional."

292.81 Amphetamine or Similarly Acting Sympathomimetic Delirium

A. Delirium (p. 77) developing within 24 hours of use of amphetamine or a similarly acting sympathomimetic.

B. Not due to any physical or other mental disorder.

Note: When the differential diagnosis must be made without a clear-cut history or toxicologic analysis of body fluids, it may be qualified as "Provisional."

292.11 Amphetamine or Similarly Acting Sympathomimetic Delusional Disorder

A. Organic Delusional Syndrome (p. 81) developing shortly after use of amphetamine or a similarly acting sympathomimetic.

B. Rapidly developing persecutory delusions are the predominant clinical feature.

C. Not due to any physical or other mental disorder.

Note: When the differential diagnosis must be made without a clear-cut history or toxicologic analysis of body fluids, it may be qualified as "Provisional."

CAFFEINE-INDUCED ORGANIC MENTAL DISORDER

305.90 Caffeine Intoxication

A. Recent consumption of caffeine, usually in excess of 250 mg.

B. At least five of the following signs:

    (1) restlessness
    (2) nervousness
    (3) excitement
    (4) insomnia
    (5) flushed face
    (6) diuresis
    (7) gastrointestinal disturbance
    (8) muscle twitching
    (9) rambling flow of thought and speech
    (10) tachycardia or cardiac arrhythmia
    (11) periods of inexhaustibility
    (12) psychomotor agitation

C. Not due to any physical or other mental disorder, such as an Anxiety Disorder.

CANNABIS-INDUCED ORGANIC MENTAL DISORDERS

305.20 Cannabis Intoxication

A. Recent use of cannabis.

B. Maladaptive behavioral changes, e.g., euphoria, anxiety, suspiciousness or paranoid ideation, sensation of slowed time, impaired judgment, social withdrawal.

C. At least two of the following signs developing within two hours of cannabis use:

(1) conjunctival injection
(2) increased appetite
(3) dry mouth
(4) tachycardia

D. Not due to any physical or other mental disorder.

Note: When the differential diagnosis must be made without a clear-cut history or toxicologic analysis of body fluids, it may be qualified as "Provisional."

292.11 Cannabis Delusional Disorder

A. Organic Delusional Syndrome (p. 81) developing shortly after cannabis use.

B. Not due to any physical or other mental disorder.

Note: When the differential diagnosis must be made without a clear-cut history or toxicologic analysis of body fluids, it may be qualified as "Provisional."

COCAINE-INDUCED ORGANIC MENTAL DISORDERS

305.60 Cocaine Intoxication

A. Recent use of cocaine.

B. Maladaptive behavioral changes, e.g., euphoria, fighting, grandiosity, hypervigilance, psychomotor agitation, impaired judgment, impaired social or occupational functioning.

C. At least two of the following signs within one hour of using cocaine:

(1) tachycardia
(2) pupillary dilation

    (3) elevated blood pressure
    (4) perspiration or chills
    (5) nausea or vomiting
    (6) visual or tactile hallucinations

D. Not due to any physical or other mental disorder.

Note: When the differential diagnosis must be made without a clear-cut history or toxicologic analysis of body fluids, it may be qualified as "Provisional."

292.00 Cocaine Withdrawal

A. Cessation of prolonged (several days or longer) heavy use of cocaine, or reduction in the amount of cocaine used, followed by dysphoric mood (e.g., depression, irritability, anxiety) and at least one of the following, persisting more than 24 hours after cessation of substance use:

    (1) fatigue
    (2) insomnia or hypersomnia
    (3) psychomotor agitation

B. Not due to any physical or other mental disorder, such as Cocaine Delusional Disorder.

Note: When the differential diagnosis must be made without a clear-cut history or toxicologic analysis of body fluids, it may be qualified as "Provisional."

292.81 Cocaine Delirium

A. Delirium (p. 77) developing within 24 hours of use of cocaine.

B. Not due to any physical or other mental disorder.

Note: When the differential diagnosis must be made without a clear-cut history or toxicologic analysis of body fluids, it may be qualified as "Provisional."

292.11 Cocaine Delusional Disorder

A. Organic Delusional Syndrome (p. 81) developing shortly after use of cocaine.

B. Rapidly developing persecutory delusions are the predominant clinical feature.

C. Not due to any physical or other mental disorder.

Note: When the differential diagnosis must be made without a clear-cut history or toxicologic analysis of body fluids, it may be qualified as "Provisional."

HALLUCINOGEN-INDUCED ORGANIC MENTAL DISORDERS

305.30 Hallucinogen Hallucinosis

A. Recent use of a hallucinogen.

B. Maladaptive behavioral changes, e.g., marked anxiety or depression, ideas of reference, fear of losing one's mind, paranoid ideation, impaired judgment, impaired social or occupational functioning.

C. Perceptual changes occurring in a state of full wakefulness and alertness, e.g., subjective intensification of perceptions, depersonalization, derealization, illusions, hallucinations, synesthesias.

D. At least two of the following signs:

(1) pupillary dilation
(2) tachycardia
(3) sweating
(4) palpitations
(5) blurring of vision
(6) tremors
(7) incoordination

E. Not due to any physical or other mental disorder.

Note: When the differential diagnosis must be made without a clear-cut history or toxicologic analysis of body fluids, it may be qualified as "Provisional."

292.11 Hallucinogen Delusional Disorder

A. Organic Delusional Syndrome (p. 81) developing shortly after hallucinogen use.

B. Not due to any physical or other mental disorder, such as Schizophrenia.

Note: When the differential diagnosis must be made without a clear-cut history or toxicologic analysis of body fluids, it may be qualified as "Provisional."

292.84 Hallucinogen Mood Disorder

A. Organic Mood Syndrome (p. 81) developing shortly after hallucinogen use (usually within one or two weeks), and persisting more than 24 hours after cessation of such use.

B. Not due to any physical or other mental disorder.

Note: When the differential diagnosis must be made without a clear-cut history or toxicologic analysis of body fluids, it may be qualified as "Provisional."

292.89 Posthallucinogen Perception Disorder

A. The reexperiencing, following cessation of use of a hallucinogen, of one or more of the perceptual symptoms that were experienced while intoxicated with the hallucinogen, e.g., geometric hallucinations, false perceptions of movement in the peripheral visual fields, flashes of color, intensified colors, trails of images from moving objects, positive afterimages, halos around objects, macropsia, and micropsia.

B. The disturbance in A causes marked distress.

C. Other causes of the symptoms, such as anatomic lesions and infections of the brain, Delirium, Dementia, sensory (visual) epilepsies, Schizophrenia, entoptic imagery, and hypnopompic hallucinations, have been ruled out.

INHALANT-INDUCED ORGANIC MENTAL DISORDER

305.90 Inhalant Intoxication

A. Recent use of an inhalant.

B. Maladaptive behavioral changes, e.g., belligerence, assaultiveness, apathy, impaired judgment, impaired social or occupational functioning.

C. At least two of the following signs:

    (1) dizziness
    (2) nystagmus
    (3) incoordination
    (4) slurred speech
    (5) unsteady gait
    (6) lethargy
    (7) depressed reflexes
    (8) psychomotor retardation
    (9) tremor
    (10) generalized muscle weakness
    (11) blurred vision or diplopia
    (12) stupor or coma
    (13) euphoria

D. Not due to any physical or other mental disorder.

Note: When the differential diagnosis must be made without a clear-cut history or toxicologic analysis of body fluids, it may be qualified as "Provisional."

NICOTINE-INDUCED ORGANIC MENTAL DISORDER

292.00 Nicotine Withdrawal

A. Daily use of nicotine for at least several weeks.

B. Abrupt cessation of nicotine use, or reduction in the amount of nicotine used, followed within 24 hours by at least four of the following signs:
   (1) craving for nicotine
   (2) irritability, frustration, or anger
   (3) anxiety
   (4) difficulty concentrating
   (5) restlessness
   (6) decreased heart rate
   (7) increased appetite or weight gain

OPIOID-INDUCED ORGANIC MENTAL DISORDERS

305.50 Opioid Intoxication

A. Recent use of an opioid.

B. Maladaptive behavioral changes, e.g., initial euphoria followed by apathy, dysphoria, psychomotor retardation, impaired judgment, impaired social or occupational functioning.

C. Pupillary constriction (or pupillary dilation due to anoxia from severe overdose) and at least one of the following signs:
   (1) drowsiness
   (2) slurred speech
   (3) impairment in attention or memory

D. Not due to any physical or other mental disorder.

Note: When the differential diagnosis must be made without a clear-cut history, testing with an opioid antagonist, or toxicologic analysis of body fluids, it may be qualified as "Provisional."

292.00 Opioid Withdrawal

A. Cessation of prolonged (several weeks or more) moderate or heavy use of an opioid, or reduction in the amount of opioid used (or administration of an opioid antagonist after a brief period of use), followed by at least three of the following:

 (1) craving for an opioid
 (2) nausea or vomiting
 (3) muscle aches
 (4) lacrimation or rhinorrhea
 (5) pupillary dilation, piloerection, or sweating
 (6) diarrhea
 (7) yawning
 (8) fever
 (9) insomnia

B. Not due to any physical or other mental disorder.

Note: When the differential diagnosis must be made without a clear-cut history or toxicologic analysis of body fluids, it may be qualified as "Provisional."

PHENCYCLIDINE (PCP)- OR SIMILARLY ACTING ARYLCYCLOHEXYLAMINE-INDUCED ORGANIC MENTAL DISORDERS

305.90 Phencyclidine (PCP) or Similarly Acting Arylcyclohexylamine Intoxication

A. Recent use of phencyclidine or a similarly acting arylcyclohexylamine.

B. Maladaptive behavioral changes, e.g., belligerence, assaultiveness, impulsiveness, unpredictability, psychomotor agitation, impaired judgment, impaired social or occupational functioning.

C. Within an hour (less when smoked, insufflated ["snorted"], or used intravenously), at least two of the following signs:

    (1) vertical or horizontal nystagmus
    (2) increased blood pressure or heart rate
    (3) numbness or diminished responsiveness to pain
    (4) ataxia
    (5) dysarthria
    (6) muscle rigidity
    (7) seizures
    (8) hyperacusis

D. Not due to any physical or other mental disorder, e.g., Phencyclidine (PCP) or Similarly Acting Arylcyclohexylamine Delirium.

Note: When the differential diagnosis must be made without a clear-cut history or toxicologic analysis of body fluids, it may be qualified as "Provisional."

292.81 Phencyclidine (PCP) or Similarly Acting Arylcyclohexylamine Delirium

A. Delirium (p. 77) developing shortly after use of phencyclidine or a similarly acting arylcyclohexylamine.

B. Not due to any physical or other mental disorder.

Note: When the differential diagnosis must be made without a clear-cut history or toxicologic analysis of body fluids, it may be qualified as "Provisional."

292.11 Phencyclidine (PCP) or Similarly Acting Arylcyclohexylamine Delusional Disorder

A. Organic Delusional Syndrome (p. 81) developing shortly after use of phencyclidine or a similarly acting arylcyclohexylamine, or emerging up to a week after an overdose.

B. Not due to any physical or other mental disorder, such as Schizophrenia.

Note: When the differential diagnosis must be made without a clear-cut history or toxicologic analysis of body fluids, it may be qualified as "Provisional."

292.84 Phencyclidine or Similarly Acting Arylcyclohexylamine Mood Disorder

A. Organic Mood Syndrome (p. 81) developing shortly after use of phencyclidine or a similarly acting arylcyclohexylamine (usually within one or two weeks) and persisting more than 24 hours after cessation of substance use.

B. Not due to any physical or other mental disorder.

Note: When the differential diagnosis must be made without a clear-cut history or toxicologic analysis of body fluids, it may be qualified as "Provisional."

292.90 Phencyclidine (PCP) or Similarly Acting Arylcyclohexylamine Organic Mental Disorder Not Otherwise Specified

A. Recent use of phencyclidine or a similarly acting arylcyclohexylamine.

B. The resulting illness involves features of several Organic Mental Syndromes or a progression from one Organic Mental Syndrome to another, e.g., initially there is Delirium, followed by an Organic Delusional Syndrome.

C. Not due to any physical or other mental disorder.

Note: When the differential diagnosis must be made without a clear-cut history or toxicologic analysis of body fluids, it may be qualified as "Provisional."

SEDATIVE-, HYPNOTIC-, OR ANXIOLYTIC-INDUCED ORGANIC MENTAL DISORDERS

305.40 Sedative, Hypnotic, or Anxiolytic Intoxication

A. Recent use of a sedative, hypnotic, or anxiolytic.

B. Maladaptive behavioral changes, e.g., disinhibition of sexual or aggressive impulses, mood lability, impaired judgment, impaired social or occupational functioning.

C. At least one of the following signs:

    (1) slurred speech
    (2) incoordination
    (3) unsteady gait
    (4) impairment in attention or memory

D. Not due to any physical or other mental disorder.

Note: When the differential diagnosis must be made without a clear-cut history or toxicologic analysis of body fluids, it may be qualified as "Provisional."

292.00 Uncomplicated Sedative, Hypnotic, or Anxiolytic Withdrawal

A. Cessation of prolonged (several weeks or more) moderate or heavy use of a sedative, hypnotic, or

anxiolytic, or reduction in the amount of substance used, followed by at least three of the following:

(1) nausea or vomiting
(2) malaise or weakness
(3) autonomic hyperactivity, e.g., tachycardia,
    sweating
(4) anxiety or irritability
(5) orthostatic hypotension
(6) coarse tremor of hands, tongue, and eyelids
(7) marked insomnia
(8) grand mal seizures

C. Not due to any physical or other mental disorder,
   such as Sedative, Hypnotic, or Anxiolytic Withdrawal Delirium.

Note: When the differential diagnosis must be made
without a clear-cut history or toxicologic analysis of
body fluids, it may be qualified as "Provisional."

292.00 Sedative, Hypnotic, or Anxiolytic Withdrawal Delirium

A. Delirium (p. 77) developing after the cessation of
   heavy use of a sedative, hypnotic, or anxiolytic, or
   a reduction in the amount of substance used (usually within one week).

B. Autonomic hyperactivity, e.g., tachycardia, sweating.

C. Not due to any physical or other mental disorder.

Note: When the differential diagnosis must be made
without a clear-cut history or toxicologic analysis of
body fluids, it may be qualified as "Provisional."

292.83 Sedative, Hypnotic, or Anxiolytic Amnestic Disorder

A. Amnestic Syndrome (p. 80) following prolonged heavy use of a sedative, hypnotic, or anxiolytic.

B. Not due to any physical or other mental disorder.

Note: When the differential diagnosis must be made without a clear-cut history or toxicologic analysis of body fluids, it may be qualified as "Provisional."

Other or Unspecified Psychoactive Substance-induced Organic Mental Disorders

These codes are to be used when a person develops an Organic Mental Syndrome apparently due to use of a psychoactive substance if:

(1) the substance cannot be classified in any of the eleven previously listed categories (*Examples:* Levo-dopa Delusional Disorder, Anticholinergic Delirium);

(2) the syndrome is caused by an unknown substance (*Example*: an intoxication after taking a bottle of unlabeled pills).

Following the listing of each of the diagnoses in this section, the reader is directed to the page listing the diagnostic criteria for the appropriate Organic Mental Syndrome.

305.90 Other or Unspecified Psychoactive Substance Intoxication (p. 83)

292.00 Other or Unspecified Psychoactive Substance Withdrawal (p. 83)

292.81 Other or Unspecified Psychoactive Substance Delirium (p. 77)

292.82 Other or Unspecified Psychoactive Substance Dementia (p. 78)

292.83 Other or Unspecified Psychoactive Substance Amnestic Disorder (p. 80)

292.11 Other or Unspecified Psychoactive Substance Delusional Disorder (p. 81)

292.12 Other or Unspecified Psychoactive Substance Hallucinosis (p. 81)

292.84 Other or Unspecified Psychoactive Substance Mood Disorder (p. 81)

292.89 Other or Unspecified Psychoactive Substance Anxiety Disorder (p. 82)

292.89 Other or Unspecified Psychoactive Substance Personality Disorder (p. 82)

292.90 Other or Unspecified Psychoactive Substance Organic Mental Disorder Not Otherwise Specified (p. 84)

ORGANIC MENTAL DISORDERS ASSOCIATED WITH AXIS III PHYSICAL DISORDERS OR CONDITIONS, OR WHOSE ETIOLOGY IS UNKNOWN

These codes permit the identification of specific Organic Mental Disorders on Axis I associated with physical disorders recorded on Axis III. Examples include Delirium (Axis I) associated with pneumonia (Axis III), and Dementia (Axis I) associated with brain tumor (Axis III). Following the name of each of the Organic Mental Disorders is the page listing the diagnostic criteria for the corresponding syndrome.

293.00 Delirium (p. 77)

294.10 Dementia (p. 78)

294.00 Amnestic Disorder (p. 80)

293.81 Organic Delusional Disorder (p. 81)

293.82 Organic Hallucinosis (p. 81)

293.83 Organic Mood Disorder (p. 82)
  Specify: manic, depressed, or mixed.

294.80 Organic Anxiety Disorder (p. 82)

310.10 Organic Personality Disorder (p. 82)
  Specify if explosive type.

294.80 Organic Mental Disorder Not Otherwise Specified (p. 84)

Psychoactive Substance Use Disorders

The following criteria are to be applied to each of the specific substances listed below.

Psychoactive Substance Dependence

A. At least three of the following:

(1) substance often taken in larger amounts or over a longer period than the person intended

(2) persistent desire or one or more unsuccessful efforts to cut down or control substance use

(3) a great deal of time spent in activities necessary to get the substance (e.g., theft), taking the substance (e.g., chain smoking), or recovering from its effects

(4) frequent intoxication or withdrawal symptoms when expected to fulfill major role obligations at work, school, or home (e.g., does not go to work because hung over, goes to school or work "high," intoxicated while taking care of his or her children), or when substance use is physically hazardous (e.g., drives when intoxicated)

(5) important social, occupational, or recreational activities given up or reduced because of substance use

(6) continued substance use despite knowledge

of having a persistent or recurrent social, psychological, or physical problem that is caused or exacerbated by the use of the substance (e.g., keeps using heroin despite family arguments about it, cocaine-induced depression, or having an ulcer made worse by drinking)

(7) marked tolerance: need for markedly increased amounts of the substance (i.e., at least a 50% increase) in order to achieve intoxication or desired effect, or markedly diminished effect with continued use of the same amount

Note: The following items may not apply to cannabis, hallucinogens, or phencyclidine (PCP):

(8) characteristic withdrawal symptoms (see specific withdrawal syndromes under Psychoactive Substance-induced Organic Mental Disorders)

(9) substance often taken to relieve or avoid withdrawal symptoms

B. Some symptoms of the disturbance have persisted for at least one month, or have occurred repeatedly over a longer period of time.

Criteria for severity of Psychoactive Substance Dependence:

Mild: Few, if any, symptoms in excess of those required to make the diagnosis, and the symptoms result in only mild impairment in occupational functioning or in usual social activities or relationships with others.

Moderate: Symptoms or functional impairment intermediate between "mild" and "severe."

Severe: Many symptoms in excess of those required to make the diagnosis, and the symptoms markedly interfere with occupational functioning or with usual social activities or relationships with others.[1]

In Partial Remission: During the past six months, some use of the substance and some symptoms of dependence.

In Full Remission: During the past six months, either no use of the substance, or use of the substance and no symptoms of dependence.

Psychoactive Substance Abuse

A. A maladaptive pattern of psychoactive substance use indicated by at least one of the following:

(1) continued use despite knowledge of having a persistent or recurrent social, occupational, psychological, or physical problem that is caused or exacerbated by use of the psychoactive substance

(2) recurrent use in situations in which use is physically hazardous (e.g., driving while intoxicated)

B. Some symptoms of the disturbance have persisted for at least one month, or have occurred repeatedly over a longer period of time.

C. Never met the criteria for Psychoactive Substance Dependence for this substance.

303.90 Alcohol Dependence
305.00 Alcohol Abuse

304.40 Amphetamine or Similarly Acting Sympathomimetic Dependence

---

[1] Because of the availability of cigarettes and other nicotine-containing substances, and the absence of a clinically significant nicotine intoxication syndrome, impairment in occupational or social functioning is not necessary for a rating of severe Nicotine Dependence.

305.70 Amphetamine or Similarly Acting Sympathomimetic Abuse

304.30 Cannabis Dependence
305.20 Cannabis Abuse

304.20 Cocaine Dependence
305.60 Cocaine Abuse

304.50 Hallucinogen Dependence
305.30 Hallucinogen Abuse

304.60 Inhalant Dependence
305.90 Inhalant Abuse

305.10 Nicotine Dependence

304.00 Opioid Dependence
305.50 Opioid Abuse

304.50 Phencyclidine (PCP) or Similarly Acting Arylcyclohexylamine Dependence
305.90 Phencyclidine (PCP) or Similarly Acting Arylcyclohexylamine Abuse

304.10 Sedative, Hypnotic, or Anxiolytic Dependence
305.40 Sedative, Hypnotic, or Anxiolytic Abuse

304.90 Polysubstance Dependence

This category should be used when, for a period of at least six months, the person has repeatedly used at least three categories of psychoactive substances (not including nicotine and caffeine), but no single psychoactive substance has predominated. During this period the criteria have been met for dependence on psychoactive substances as a group, but not for any specific substance.

304.90 Psychoactive Substance Dependence Not Otherwise Specified

This is a residual category for disorders in which there is dependence on a psychoactive substance that cannot be classified according to any of the previous categories (e.g., anticholinergics), or for use as an initial diagnosis in cases of dependence in which the specific substance is not yet known.

305.90 Psychoactive Substance Abuse Not Otherwise Specified

This is a residual category for disorders in which there is abuse of a psychoactive substance that cannot be classified in any of the previous categories (e.g., anticholinergics), or for use as an initial diagnosis in cases of abuse in which the specific substance is not yet known.

Schizophrenia

295.xx Schizophrenia

A. Presence of characteristic psychotic symptoms in the active phase: either (1), (2), or (3) for at least one week (unless the symptoms are successfully treated):

(1) two of the following:

   (a) delusions
   (b) prominent hallucinations (throughout the day for several days or several times a week for several weeks, each hallucinatory experience not being limited to a few brief moments)
   (c) incoherence or marked loosening of associations
   (d) catatonic behavior
   (e) flat or grossly inappropriate affect

(2) bizarre delusions (i.e., involving a phenomenon that the person's culture would regard as totally implausible, e.g., thought broadcasting, being controlled by a dead person)

(3) prominent hallucinations (as defined in [1b] above) of a voice with content having no apparent relation to depression or elation, or a voice keeping up a running commentary on

the person's behavior or thoughts, or two or more voices conversing with each other

B. During the course of the disturbance, functioning in such areas as work, social relations, and self-care is markedly below the highest level achieved before onset of the disturbance (or, when the onset is in childhood or adolescence, failure to achieve expected level of social development).

C. Schizoaffective Disorder and Mood Disorder with Psychotic Features have been ruled out, i.e., if a Major Depressive or Manic Syndrome has ever been present during an active phase of the disturbance, the total duration of all episodes of a mood syndrome has been brief relative to the total duration of the active and residual phases of the disturbance.

D. Continuous signs of the disturbance for at least six months. The six-month period must include an active phase (of at least one week, or less if symptoms have been successfully treated) during which there were psychotic symptoms characteristic of Schizophrenia (symptoms in A), with or without a prodromal or residual phase, as defined below.

Prodromal phase: A clear deterioration in functioning before the active phase of the disturbance that is not due to a disturbance in mood or to a Psychoactive Substance Use Disorder and that involves at least two of the symptoms listed below.

Residual phase: Following the active phase of the disturbance, persistence of at least two of the symptoms noted below, these not being due to a disturbance in mood or to a Psychoactive Substance Use Disorder.

Prodromal or Residual Symptoms:

(1) marked social isolation or withdrawal
(2) marked impairment in role functioning as wage-earner, student, or homemaker
(3) markedly peculiar behavior (e.g., collecting garbage, talking to self in public, hoarding food)
(4) marked impairment in personal hygiene and grooming
(5) blunted or inappropriate affect
(6) digressive, vague, overelaborate, or circumstantial speech, or poverty of speech, or poverty of content of speech
(7) odd beliefs or magical thinking, influencing behavior and inconsistent with cultural norms, e.g., superstitiousness, belief in clairvoyance, telepathy, "sixth sense," "others can feel my feelings," overvalued ideas, ideas of reference
(8) unusual perceptual experiences, e.g., recurrent illusions, sensing the presence of a force or person not actually present
(9) marked lack of initiative, interests, or energy

Examples: Six months of prodromal symptoms with one week of symptoms from A; no prodromal symptoms with six months of symptoms from A; no prodromal symptoms with one week of symptoms from A and six months of residual symptoms.

E. It cannot be established that an organic factor initiated and maintained the disturbance.

F. If there is a history of Autistic Disorder, the additional diagnosis of Schizophrenia is made only if prominent delusions or hallucinations are also present.

Classification of course. The course of the disturbance is coded in the fifth digit:

1-Subchronic. The time from the beginning of the disturbance, when the person first began to show signs of the disturbance (including prodromal, active, and residual phases) more or less continuously, is less than two years, but at least six months.

2-Chronic. Same as above, but more than two years.

3-Subchronic with Acute Exacerbation. Reemergence of prominent psychotic symptoms in a person with a subchronic course who has been in the residual phase of the disturbance.

4-Chronic with Acute Exacerbation. Reemergence of prominent psychotic symptoms in a person with a chronic course who has been in the residual phase of the disturbance.

5-In Remission. When a person with a history of Schizophrenia is free of all signs of the disturbance (whether or not on medication), "in Remission" should be coded. Differentiating Schizophrenia in Remission from No Mental Disorder requires consideration of overall level of functioning, length of time since the last episode of disturbance, total duration of the disturbance, and whether prophylactic treatment is being given.

0-Unspecified.

When the course is noted as "in Remission," the phenomenologic type should describe the last exacerbation of Schizophrenia, e.g., "295.25 Schizophrenia, Catatonic Type, in Remission." When the phenomenology of the last exacerbation is unknown, it should be noted as "Undifferentiated."

Specify late onset if the disturbance (including the prodromal phase) develops after age 45.

Types

The diagnosis of a particular type should be based on the predominant clinical picture that occasioned the most recent evaluation or admission to clinical care.

295.2x Catatonic Type

A type of Schizophrenia in which the clinical picture is dominated by any of the following:

(1) catatonic stupor (marked decrease in reactivity to the environment and/or reduction in spontaneous movements and activity) or mutism

(2) catatonic negativism (an apparently motiveless resistance to all instructions or attempts to be moved)

(3) catatonic rigidity (maintenance of a rigid posture against efforts to be moved)

(4) catatonic excitement (excited motor activity, apparently purposeless and not influenced by external stimuli)

(5) catatonic posturing (voluntary assumption of inappropriate or bizarre postures)

295.1x Disorganized Type

A type of Schizophrenia in which the following criteria are met:

A. Incoherence, marked loosening of associations, or grossly disorganized behavior.

B. Flat or grossly inappropriate affect.

C. Does not meet the criteria for Catatonic Type.

295.3x Paranoid Type

A type of Schizophrenia in which there are:

A. Preoccupation with one or more systematized delusions or with frequent auditory hallucinations related to a single theme.

B. *None* of the following: incoherence, marked loosening of associations, flat or grossly inappropriate affect, catatonic behavior, grossly disorganized behavior.

Specify stable type if criteria A and B have been met during all past and present active phases of the illness.

295.9x Undifferentiated Type

A type of Schizophrenia in which there are:

A. Prominent delusions, hallucinations, incoherence, or grossly disorganized behavior.

B. Does not meet the criteria for Paranoid, Catatonic, or Disorganized Type.

295.6x Residual Type

A type of Schizophrenia in which there are:

A. Absence of prominent delusions, hallucinations, incoherence, or grossly disorganized behavior.

B. Continuing evidence of the disturbance, as indicated by two or more of the residual symptoms listed in criterion D of Schizophrenia.

Delusional (Paranoid) Disorder

297.10 Delusional (Paranoid) Disorder

A. Nonbizarre delusion(s) (i.e., involving situations that occur in real life, such as being followed, poisoned, infected, loved at a distance, having a disease, being deceived by one's spouse or lover) of at least one month's duration.

B. Auditory or visual hallucinations, if present, are not prominent (as defined in Schizophrenia, A[1*b*]).

C. Apart from the delusion(s) or its ramifications, behavior is not obviously odd or bizarre.

D. If a Major Depressive or Manic Syndrome has been present during the delusional disturbance, the total duration of all episodes of the mood syndrome has been brief relative to the total duration of the delusional disturbance.

E. Has never met criterion A for Schizophrenia, and it cannot be established that an organic factor initiated and maintained the disturbance.

Specify type: The following types are based on the predominant delusional theme. If no single delusional theme predominates, specify as **Unspecified Type.**

Erotomanic Type

Delusional Disorder in which the predominant theme of the delusion(s) is that a person, usually of higher status, is in love with the subject.

Grandiose Type

Delusional Disorder in which the predominant theme of the delusion(s) is one of inflated worth, power, knowledge, identity, or special relationship to a deity or famous person.

Jealous Type

Delusional Disorder in which the predominant theme of the delusion(s) is that one's sexual partner is unfaithful.

Persecutory Type

Delusional Disorder in which the predominant theme of the delusion(s) is that one (or someone to whom one is close) is being malevolently treated in some way. People with this type of Delusional Disorder may repeatedly take their complaints of being mistreated to legal authorities.

Somatic Type

Delusional Disorder in which the predominant theme of the delusion(s) is that the person has some physical defect, disorder, or disease.

Unspecified Type

Delusional Disorder that does not fit any of the previous categories, e.g., persecutory and grandiose themes without a predominance of either; delusions of reference without malevolent content.

Psychotic Disorders Not Elsewhere Classified

298.80 Brief Reactive Psychosis

A. Presence of at least one of the following symptoms indicating impaired reality testing (not culturally sanctioned):

   (1) incoherence or marked loosening of associations
   (2) delusions
   (3) hallucinations
   (4) catatonic or disorganized behavior

B. Emotional turmoil, i.e., rapid shifts from one intense affect to another, or overwhelming perplexity or confusion.

C. Appearance of the symptoms in A and B shortly after, and apparently in response to, one or more events that, singly or together, would be markedly stressful to almost anyone in similar circumstances in the person's culture.

D. Absence of the prodromal symptoms of Schizophrenia, and failure to meet the criteria for Schizotypal Personality Disorder before onset of the disturbance.

E. Duration of an episode of the disturbance of from a few hours to one month, with eventual full return to premorbid level of functioning. (When the diagnosis must be made without waiting for the expected recovery, it should be qualified as "provisional.")

F. Not due to a psychotic Mood Disorder (i.e., no full mood syndrome is present), and it cannot be established that an organic factor initiated and maintained the disturbance.

295.40 Schizophreniform Disorder

A. Meets criteria A and C of Schizophrenia (p. 113 and 114).

B. An episode of the disturbance (including prodromal, active, and residual phases) lasts less than six months. (When the diagnosis must be made without waiting for recovery, it should be qualified as "provisional.")

C. Does not meet the criteria for Brief Reactive Psychosis, and it cannot be established that an organic factor initiated and maintained the disturbance.

Specify: without good prognostic features or

with good prognostic features, i.e., with at least two of the following:

(1) onset of prominent psychotic symptoms within four weeks of first noticeable change in usual behavior or functioning
(2) confusion, disorientation, or perplexity at the height of the psychotic episode
(3) good premorbid social and occupational functioning
(4) absence of blunted or flat affect

295.70 Schizoaffective Disorder

A. A disturbance during which, at some time, there is either a Major Depressive or a Manic Syndrome concurrent with symptoms that meet the A criterion of Schizophrenia.

B. During an episode of the disturbance, there have been delusions or hallucinations for at least two weeks, but no prominent mood symptoms.

C. Schizophrenia has been ruled out, i.e., the duration of all episodes of a mood syndrome has not been brief relative to the total duration of the psychotic disturbance.

D. It cannot be established that an organic factor initiated and maintained the disturbance.

Specify: **bipolar type** (current or previous Manic Syndrome) or

depressive type (no current or previous Manic Syndrome)

297.30 Induced Psychotic Disorder (Shared Paranoid Disorder)

A. A delusion develops (in a second person) in the context of a close relationship with another person, or persons, with an already established delusion (the primary case).

B. The delusion in the second person is similar in content to that in the primary case.

C. Immediately before onset of the induced delusion, the second person did not have a psychotic disorder or the prodromal symptoms of Schizophrenia.

298.90 Psychotic Disorder Not Otherwise Specified (Atypical Psychosis)

Disorders in which there are psychotic symptoms (delusions, hallucinations, incoherence, marked loosening of associations, catatonic excitement or stupor, or grossly disorganized behavior) that do not meet the criteria for any other nonorganic psychotic disorder. This category should also be used for psychoses about which there is inadequate information to make a specific diagnosis. (This is preferable to "Diagnosis Deferred," and can be changed if more information becomes available.) This diagnosis is made only when it cannot be established that an organic factor initiated and maintained the disturbance.

Examples:

(1) psychoses with unusual features, e.g., persistent auditory hallucinations as the only disturbance
(2) postpartum psychoses that do not meet the criteria for an Organic Mental Disorder, psychotic Mood Disorder, or any other psychotic disorder
(3) psychoses with confusing clinical features that make a more specific diagnosis impossible

Mood Disorders

In this section, criteria are provided for Manic and Major Depressive Episodes. These are followed by criteria for the specific mood disorders.

Manic Episode

Note: A "Manic Syndrome" is defined as including criteria A, B, and C below. A "Hypomanic Syndrome" is defined as including criteria A and B, but not C, i.e., no marked impairment.

A. A distinct period of abnormally and persistently elevated, expansive, or irritable mood.

B. During the period of mood disturbance, at least three of the following symptoms have persisted (four if the mood is only irritable) and have been present to a significant degree:

   (1) inflated self-esteem or grandiosity
   (2) decreased need for sleep, e.g., feels rested after only three hours of sleep
   (3) more talkative than usual or pressure to keep talking
   (4) flight of ideas or subjective experience that thoughts are racing
   (5) distractibility, i.e., attention too easily drawn to unimportant or irrelevant external stimuli

(6) increase in goal-directed activity (either socially, at work or school, or sexually) or psychomotor agitation

(7) excessive involvement in pleasurable activities which have a high potential for painful consequences, e.g., the person engages in unrestrained buying sprees, sexual indiscretions, or foolish business investments

C. Mood disturbance sufficiently severe to cause marked impairment in occupational functioning or in usual social activities or relationships with others, or to necessitate hospitalization to prevent harm to self or others.

D. At no time during the disturbance have there been delusions or hallucinations for as long as two weeks in the absence of prominent mood symptoms (i.e., before the mood symptoms developed or after they have remitted).

E. Not superimposed on Schizophrenia, Schizophreniform Disorder, Delusional Disorder, or Psychotic Disorder NOS.

F. It cannot be established that an organic factor initiated and maintained the disturbance. **Note:** Somatic antidepressant treatment (e.g., drugs, ECT) that apparently precipitates a mood disturbance should not be considered an etiologic organic factor.

Manic Episode codes: fifth-digit code numbers and criteria for severity of current state of Bipolar Disorder, Manic or Mixed:

1–Mild: Meets minimum symptom criteria for a Manic Episode (or almost meets symptom criteria if there has been a previous Manic Episode).

2–Moderate: Extreme increase in activity or impairment in judgment.

3–Severe, without Psychotic Features: Almost continual supervision required in order to prevent physical harm to self or others.

4–With Psychotic Features: Delusions, hallucinations, or catatonic symptoms. If possible, **specify** whether the psychotic features are *mood-congruent* or *mood-incongruent*.

Mood-congruent psychotic features: Delusions or hallucinations whose content is entirely consistent with the typical manic themes of inflated worth, power, knowledge, identity, or special relationship to a deity or famous person.

Mood-incongruent psychotic features: Either (*a*) or (*b*):

(*a*) Delusions or hallucinations whose content does *not* involve the typical manic themes of inflated worth, power, knowledge, identity, or special relationship to a deity or famous person. Included are such symptoms as persecutory delusions (not directly related to grandiose ideas or themes), thought insertion, and delusions of being controlled.

(*b*) Catatonic symptoms, e.g., stupor, mutism, negativism, posturing.

5–In Partial Remission: Full criteria were previously, but are not currently, met; some signs or symptoms of the disturbance have persisted.

6–In Full Remission: Full criteria were previously met, but there have been no significant signs or symptoms of the disturbance for at least six months.

0–Unspecified.

Major Depressive Episode

Note: A "Major Depressive Syndrome" is defined as criterion A below.

A. At least five of the following symptoms have been present during the same two-week period and represent a change from previous functioning; at least one of the symptoms is either (1) depressed mood, or (2) loss of interest or pleasure. (Do not include symptoms that are clearly due to a physical condition, mood-incongruent delusions or hallucinations, incoherence, or marked loosening of associations.)

  (1) depressed mood (or can be irritable mood in children and adolescents) most of the day, nearly every day, as indicated either by subjective account or observation by others

  (2) markedly diminished interest or pleasure in all, or almost all, activities most of the day, nearly every day (as indicated either by subjective account or observation by others of apathy most of the time)

  (3) significant weight loss or weight gain when not dieting (e.g., more than 5% of body weight in a month), or decrease or increase in appetite nearly every day (in children, consider failure to make expected weight gains)

  (4) insomnia or hypersomnia nearly every day

  (5) psychomotor agitation or retardation nearly every day (observable by others, not merely subjective feelings of restlessness or being slowed down)

  (6) fatigue or loss of energy nearly every day

  (7) feelings of worthlessness or excessive or inappropriate guilt (which may be delusional) nearly every day (not merely self-reproach or guilt about being sick)

    (8) diminished ability to think or concentrate, or indecisiveness, nearly every day (either by subjective account or as observed by others)

    (9) recurrent thoughts of death (not just fear of dying), recurrent suicidal ideation without a specific plan, or a suicide attempt or a specific plan for committing suicide

B. (1) It cannot be established that an organic factor initiated and maintained the disturbance

    (2) The disturbance is not a normal reaction to the death of a loved one (Uncomplicated Bereavement)

Note: Morbid preoccupation with worthlessness, suicidal ideation, marked functional impairment or psychomotor retardation, or prolonged duration suggest bereavement complicated by Major Depression.

C. At no time during the disturbance have there been delusions or hallucinations for as long as two weeks in the absence of prominent mood symptoms (i.e., before the mood symptoms developed or after they have remitted).

D. Not superimposed on Schizophrenia, Schizophreniform Disorder, Delusional Disorder, or Psychotic Disorder NOS.

Major depressive episode codes: fifth-digit code numbers and criteria for severity of current state of Bipolar Disorder, Depressed, or Major Depression:

1–Mild: Few, if any, symptoms in excess of those required to make the diagnosis, **and** symptoms result in only minor impairment in occupational functioning or in usual social activities or relationships with others.

2–Moderate: Symptoms or functional impairment between "mild" and "severe."

3–Severe, without Psychotic Features: Several symptoms in excess of those required to make the diagnosis, **and** symptoms markedly interfere with occupational functioning or with usual social activities or relationships with others.

4–With Psychotic Features: Delusions or hallucinations. If possible, **specify** whether the psychotic features are *mood-congruent* or *mood-incongruent.*

Mood-congruent psychotic features: Delusions or hallucinations whose content is entirely consistent with the typical depressive themes of personal inadequacy, guilt, disease, death, nihilism, or deserved punishment.

Mood-incongruent psychotic features: Delusions or hallucinations whose content does *not* involve typical depressive themes of personal inadequacy, guilt, disease, death, nihilism, or deserved punishment. Included here are such symptoms as persecutory delusions (not directly related to depressive themes), thought insertion, thought broadcasting, and delusions of control.

5–In Partial Remission: Intermediate between "In Full Remission" and "Mild," **and** no previous Dysthymia. (If Major Depressive Episode was superimposed on Dysthymia, the diagnosis of Dysthymia alone is given once the full criteria for a Major Depressive Episode are no longer met.)

6–In Full Remission: During the past six months no significant signs or symptoms of the disturbance.

0–Unspecified.

Specify chronic if current episode has lasted two consecutive years without a period of two months or longer during which there were no significant depressive symptoms.

Specify if current episode is **Melancholic Type.**

Diagnostic criteria for Melancholic Type

The presence of at least five of the following:

(1) loss of interest or pleasure in all, or almost all, activities

(2) lack of reactivity to usually pleasurable stimuli (does not feel much better, even temporarily, when something good happens)

(3) depression regularly worse in the morning

(4) early morning awakening (at least two hours before usual time of awakening)

(5) psychomotor retardation or agitation (not merely subjective complaints)

(6) significant anorexia or weight loss (e.g., more than 5% of body weight in a month)

(7) no significant personality disturbance before first major depressive episode

(8) one or more previous major depressive episodes followed by complete, or nearly complete, recovery

(9) previous good response to specific and adequate somatic antidepressant therapy, e.g., tricyclics, ECT, MAOI, lithium

Diagnostic criteria for seasonal pattern

A. There has been a regular temporal relationship between the onset of an episode of Bipolar Disorder (including Bipolar Disorder NOS) or Recurrent Major Depression (including Depressive Disorder

NOS) and a particular 60-day period of the year (e.g., regular appearance of depression between the beginning of October and the end of November).

Note: Do not include cases in which there is an obvious effect of seasonally related psychosocial stressors, e.g., regularly being unemployed every winter.

B. Full remissions (or a change from depression to mania or hypomania) also occurred within a particular 60-day period of the year (e.g., depression disappears from mid-February to mid-April).

C. There have been at least three episodes of mood disturbance in three separate years that demonstrated the temporal seasonal relationship defined in A and B; at least two of the years were consecutive.

D. Seasonal episodes of mood disturbance, as described above, outnumbered any nonseasonal episodes of such disturbance that may have occurred by more than three to one.

BIPOLAR DISORDERS

296.6x Bipolar Disorder, Mixed

For fifth digit, use the Manic Episode codes (p. 126) to describe current state.

A. Current (or most recent) episode involves the full symptomatic picture of both Manic and Major Depressive Episodes (except for the duration requirement of two weeks for depressive symptoms)

(p. 125 and p. 128), intermixed or rapidly alternating every few days.

B. Prominent depressive symptoms lasting at least a full day.

Specify if **seasonal pattern** (see p. 131).

296.4x Bipolar Disorder, Manic

For fifth digit, use the Manic Episode codes (p. 126) to describe current state.

Currently (or most recently) in a Manic Episode (p. 125). (If there has been a previous Manic Episode, the current episode need not meet the full criteria for a manic episode.)

Specify if **seasonal pattern** (see p. 131).

296.5x Bipolar Disorder, Depressed

For fifth digit, use the Major Depressive Episode codes (p. 129) to describe current state.

A. Has had one or more Manic Episodes (p. 125).

B. Currently (or most recently) in a Major Depressive Episode (p. 128). (If there has been a previous Major Depressive Episode, the current episode need not meet the full criteria for a Major Depressive Episode.)

Specify if **seasonal pattern** (see p. 131).

301.13 Cyclothymia

A. For at least two years (one year for children and adolescents), presence of numerous Hypomanic

Episodes (all of the criteria for a Manic Episode, p. 125, except criterion C that indicates marked impairment) and numerous periods with depressed mood or loss of interest or pleasure that did not meet criterion A of Major Depressive Episode.

B. During a two-year period (one year in children and adolescents) of the disturbance, never without hypomanic or depressive symptoms for more than two months at a time.

C. No clear evidence of a Major Depressive Episode or Manic Episode during the first two years of the disturbance (or one year in children and adolescents).

Note: After this minimum period of Cyclothymia, there may be superimposed Manic or Major Depressive Episodes, in which case the additional diagnosis of Bipolar Disorder or Bipolar Disorder NOS should be given.

D. Not superimposed on a chronic psychotic disorder, such as Schizophrenia or Delusional Disorder.

E. It cannot be established that an organic factor initiated and maintained the disturbance, e.g., repeated intoxication from drugs or alcohol.

296.70 Bipolar Disorder Not Otherwise Specified

Disorders with manic or hypomanic features that do not meet the criteria for any specific Bipolar Disorder.

Examples:

(1) at least one Hypomanic Episode and at least one Major Depressive Episode, but never either a Manic Episode or Cyclothymia. Such

cases have been referred to as "Bipolar II."
(2) one or more Hypomanic Episodes, but without Cyclothymia or a history of either a Manic or a Major Depressive Episode
(3) a Manic Episode superimposed on Delusional Disorder, residual Schizophrenia, or Psychotic Disorder NOS

Specify if **seasonal pattern** (see p. 131).

DEPRESSIVE DISORDERS

296.2x Major Depression, Single Episode

For fifth digit, use the Major Depressive Episode codes (p. 129) to describe current state.

A. A single Major Depressive Episode (p. 128).

B. Has never had a Manic Episode or an unequivocal Hypomanic Episode (see p. 125).

Specify if **seasonal pattern** (see p. 131).

296.3x Major Depression, Recurrent

For fifth digit, use the Major Depressive Episode codes (p. 129) to describe current state.

A. Two or more Major Depressive Episodes (p. 128), each separated by at least two months of return to more or less usual functioning. (If there has been a previous Major Depressive Episode, the current episode of depression need not meet the full criteria for a Major Depressive Episode.)

B. Has never had a Manic Episode or an unequivocal Hypomanic Episode (see p. 125).

Specify if **seasonal pattern** (see p. 131).

300.40 Dysthymia (or Depressive Neurosis)

A. Depressed mood (or can be irritable mood in children and adolescents) for most of the day, more days than not, as indicated either by subjective account or observation by others, for at least two years (one year for children and adolescents)

B. Presence, while depressed, of at least two of the following:

    (1) poor appetite or overeating
    (2) insomnia or hypersomnia
    (3) low energy or fatigue
    (4) low self-esteem
    (5) poor concentration or difficulty making decisions
    (6) feelings of hopelessness

C. During a two-year period (one-year for children and adolescents) of the disturbance, never without the symptoms in A for more than two months at a time.

D. No evidence of an unequivocal Major Depressive Episode during the first two years (one year for children and adolescents) of the disturbance.

Note: There may have been a previous Major Depressive Episode, provided there was a full remission (no significant signs or symptoms for six months) before development of the Dysthymia. In addition, after these two years (one year in children or adolescents) of Dysthymia, there may be superimposed episodes of Major Depression, in which case both diagnoses are given.

E. Has never had a Manic Episode or an unequivocal Hypomanic Episode (see p. 125).

F. Not superimposed on a chronic psychotic disorder, such as Schizophrenia or Delusional Disorder.

G. It cannot be established that an organic factor initiated and maintained the disturbance, e.g., prolonged administration of an antihypertensive medication.

Specify primary or **secondary type:**

Primary type: the mood disturbance is not related to a preexisting, chronic, nonmood Axis I or Axis III disorder, e.g., Anorexia Nervosa, Somatization Disorder, a Psychoactive Substance Dependence Disorder, an Anxiety Disorder, or rheumatoid arthritis.

Secondary type: the mood disturbance is apparently related to a preexisting, chronic, nonmood Axis I or Axis III disorder.

Specify early onset or **late onset:**

Early onset: onset of the disturbance before age 21.

Late onset: onset of the disturbance at age 21 or later.

311.00 Depressive Disorder Not Otherwise Specified

Disorders with depressive features that do not meet the criteria for any specific Mood Disorder or Adjustment Disorder with Depressed Mood.

Examples:

(1) Major Depressive Episode superimposed on residual Schizophrenia

    (2) recurrent mild depressive disturbance that does not meet the criteria for Dysthymia

    (3) non-stress-related depressive episodes that do not meet the criteria for a Major Depressive Episode

Specify if **seasonal pattern** (see p. 131).

Anxiety Disorders
(or Anxiety and Phobic Neuroses)

Panic Disorder (with and without Agoraphobia)

A. At some time during the disturbance, one or more panic attacks (discrete periods of intense fear or discomfort) have occurred that were (1) unexpected, i.e., did not occur immediately before or on exposure to a situation that almost always caused anxiety, and (2) not triggered by situations in which the person was the focus of others' attention.

B. Either four attacks, as defined in criterion A, have occurred within a four-week period, or one or more attacks have been followed by a period of at least a month of persistent fear of having another attack.

C. At least four of the following symptoms developed during at least one of the attacks:

   (1) shortness of breath (dyspnea) or smothering sensations
   (2) dizziness, unsteady feelings, or faintness
   (3) palpitations or accelerated heart rate (tachycardia)
   (4) trembling or shaking
   (5) sweating
   (6) choking
   (7) nausea or abdominal distress

  (8) depersonalization or derealization
  (9) numbness or tingling sensations (paresthesias)
(10) flushes (hot flashes) or chills
(11) chest pain or discomfort
(12) fear of dying
(13) fear of going crazy or of doing something uncontrolled

Note: Attacks involving four or more symptoms are panic attacks; attacks involving fewer than four symptoms are limited symptom attacks (see Agoraphobia without History of Panic Disorder, p. 142).

D. During at least some of the attacks, at least four of the C symptoms developed suddenly and increased in intensity within ten minutes of the beginning of the first C symptom noticed in the attack.

E. It cannot be established that an organic factor initiated and maintained the disturbance, e.g., Amphetamine or Caffeine Intoxication, hyperthyroidism.

Note: Mitral valve prolapse may be an associated condition, but does not preclude a diagnosis of Panic Disorder.

Subtypes of Panic Disorder

300.21 with agoraphobia

A. Meets the criteria for Panic Disorder.

B. Agoraphobia: Fear of being in places or situations from which escape might be difficult (or embarrassing) or in which help might not be available in the event of a panic attack. (Include cases in which persistent avoidance behavior originated during an active phase of Panic Disorder, even if the person does not attribute the avoidance behavior to fear of having a panic attack.) As a result of this fear, the person either restricts travel or needs a companion when away from home, or else endures agoraphobic situations despite intense anxiety. Common agoraphobic situations include being outside the home alone, being in a crowd or standing in a line, being on a bridge, and traveling in a bus, train, or car.

Specify current severity of agoraphobic avoidance:

Mild: Some avoidance (or endurance with distress), but relatively normal life-style, e.g., travels unaccompanied when necessary, such as to work or to shop; otherwise avoids traveling alone.

Moderate: Avoidance results in constricted life-style, e.g., the person is able to leave the house alone, but not to go more than a few miles unaccompanied.

Severe: Avoidance results in being nearly or completely housebound or unable to leave the house unaccompanied.

In Partial Remission: No current agoraphobic avoidance, but some agoraphobic avoidance during the past six months.

In Full Remission: No current agoraphobic avoidance and none during the past six months.

Specify current severity of panic attacks:

Mild: During the past month, either all attacks have been limited symptom attacks (i.e., fewer than four symptoms), or there has been no more than one panic attack.

Moderate: During the past month attacks have been intermediate between "mild" and "severe."

Severe: During the past month, there have been at least eight panic attacks.

In Partial Remission: The condition has been intermediate between "In Full Remission" and "Mild."

In Full Remission: During the past six months, there have been no panic or limited symptom attacks.

300.01 without agoraphobia

A. Meets the criteria for Panic Disorder.

B. Absence of Agoraphobia, as defined above.

Specify current severity of panic attacks, as defined above.

300.22 Agoraphobia without History of Panic Disorder

A. Agoraphobia: Fear of being in places or situations from which escape might be difficult (or embarrassing) or in which help might not be available in the event of suddenly developing a symptom(s) that could be incapacitating or extremely embarrassing. Examples include: dizziness or falling, depersonalization or derealization, loss of bladder or bowel control, vomiting, or cardiac distress. As a result of this fear, the person either restricts travel or needs a companion when away from home, or else endures agoraphobic situations despite intense anxiety. Common agoraphobic situations include being outside the home alone, being in a crowd or standing in a line, being on a bridge, and traveling in a bus, train, or car.

B. Has never met the criteria for Panic Disorder.

Specify with or **without limited symptom attacks (see p. 140).**

300.23 Social Phobia

A. A persistent fear of one or more situations (the social phobic situations) in which the person is exposed to possible scrutiny by others and fears that he or she may do something or act in a way that will be humiliating or embarrassing. Examples include: being unable to continue talking while speaking in public, choking on food when eating in front of others, being unable to urinate in a public lavatory, hand-trembling when writing in the presence of others, and saying foolish things or not being able to answer questions in social situations.

B. If an Axis III or another Axis I disorder is present, the fear in A is unrelated to it, e.g., the fear is not of having a panic attack (Panic Disorder), stuttering (Stuttering), trembling (Parkinson's disease), or exhibiting abnormal eating behavior (Anorexia Nervosa or Bulimia Nervosa).

C. During some phase of the disturbance, exposure to the specific phobic stimulus (or stimuli) almost invariably provokes an immediate anxiety response.

D. The phobic situation(s) is avoided, or is endured with intense anxiety.

E. The avoidant behavior interferes with occupational functioning or with usual social activities or relationships with others, or there is marked distress about having the fear.

F. The person recognizes that his or her fear is excessive or unreasonable.

G. If the person is under 18, the disturbance does not
    meet the criteria for Avoidant Disorder of Child-
    hood or Adolescence.

Specify generalized type if the phobic situation includes most social situations, and also consider the
additional diagnosis of Avoidant Personality Disorder.

300.29 Simple Phobia

A. A persistent fear of a circumscribed stimulus (ob-
    ject or situation) other than fear of having a panic
    attack (as in Panic Disorder) or of humiliation or
    embarrassment in certain social situations (as in
    Social Phobia).

    Note: Do not include fears that are part of Panic
    Disorder with Agoraphobia or Agoraphobia with-
    out History of Panic Disorder.

B. During some phase of the disturbance, exposure
    to the specific phobic stimulus (or stimuli) almost
    invariably provokes an immediate anxiety re-
    sponse.

C. The object or situation is avoided, or endured with
    intense anxiety.

D. The fear or the avoidant behavior significantly in-
    terferes with the person's normal routine or with
    usual social activities or relationships with others,
    or there is marked distress about having the fear.

E. The person recognizes that his or her fear is exces-
    sive or unreasonable.

F. The phobic stimulus is unrelated to the content of
    the obsessions of Obsessive Compulsive Disorder
    or the trauma of Post-traumatic Stress Disorder.

300.30 Obsessive Compulsive Disorder
(or Obsessive Compulsive Neurosis)

A. Either obsessions or compulsions:

Obsessions: (1), (2), (3), and (4):

(1) recurrent and persistent ideas, thoughts, impulses, or images that are experienced, at least initially, as intrusive and senseless, e.g., a parent's having repeated impulses to kill loved child, a religious person's having recurrent blasphemous thoughts

(2) the person attempts to ignore or suppress such thoughts or impulses or to neutralize them with some other thought or action

(3) the person recognizes that the obsessions are the product of his or her own mind, not imposed from without (as in thought insertion)

(4) if another Axis I disorder is present, the content of the obsession is unrelated to it, e.g., the ideas, thoughts, impulses, or images are not about food in the presence of an Eating Disorder, about drugs in the presence of a Psychoactive Substance Use Disorder, or guilty thoughts in the presence of a Major Depression

Compulsions: (1), (2), and (3):

(1) repetitive, purposeful, and intentional behaviors that are performed in response to an obsession, or according to certain rules or in a stereotyped fashion

(2) the behavior is designed to neutralize or to prevent discomfort or some dreaded event or situation; however, either the activity is not connected in a realistic way with what it is

designed to neutralize or prevent, or it is clearly excessive

(3) the person recognizes that his or her behavior is excessive or unreasonable (this may not be true for young children; it may no longer be true for people whose obsessions have evolved into overvalued ideas)

B. The obsessions or compulsions cause marked distress, are time-consuming (take more than an hour a day), or significantly interfere with the person's normal routine, occupational functioning, or usual social activities or relationships with others.

309.89 Post-traumatic Stress Disorder

A. The person has experienced an event that is outside the range of usual human experience and that would be markedly distressing to almost anyone, e.g., serious threat to one's life or physical integrity; serious threat or harm to one's children, spouse, or other close relatives and friends; sudden destruction of one's home or community; or seeing another person who has recently been, or is being, seriously injured or killed as the result of an accident or physical violence.

B. The traumatic event is persistently reexperienced in at least one of the following ways:

(1) recurrent and intrusive distressing recollections of the event (in young children, repetitive play in which themes or aspects of the trauma are expressed)

(2) recurrent distressing dreams of the event

(3) sudden acting or feeling as if the traumatic event were recurring (includes a sense of reliv-

ing the experience, illusions, hallucinations, and dissociative [flashback] episodes, even those that occur upon awakening or when intoxicated)

(4) intense psychological distress at exposure to events that symbolize or resemble an aspect of the traumatic event, including anniversaries of the trauma

C. Persistent avoidance of stimuli associated with the trauma or numbing of general responsiveness (not present before the trauma), as indicated by at least three of the following:

(1) efforts to avoid thoughts or feelings associated with the trauma

(2) efforts to avoid activities or situations that arouse recollections of the trauma

(3) inability to recall an important aspect of the trauma (psychogenic amnesia)

(4) markedly diminished interest in significant activities (in young children, loss of recently acquired developmental skills such as toilet training or language skills)

(5) feeling of detachment or estrangement from others

(6) restricted range of affect, e.g., unable to have loving feelings

(7) sense of a foreshortened future, e.g., does not expect to have a career, marriage, or children, or a long life

D. Persistent symptoms of increased arousal (not present before the trauma), as indicated by at least two of the following:

(1) difficulty falling or staying asleep

    (2) irritability or outbursts of anger
    (3) difficulty concentrating
    (4) hypervigilance
    (5) exaggerated startle response
    (6) physiologic reactivity upon exposure to events that symbolize or resemble an aspect of the traumatic event (e.g., a woman who was raped in an elevator breaks out in a sweat when entering any elevator)

E. Duration of the disturbance (symptoms in B, C, and D) of at least one month.

Specify delayed onset if the onset of symptoms was at least six months after the trauma.

300.02 Generalized Anxiety Disorder

A. Unrealistic or excessive anxiety and worry (apprehensive expectation) about two or more life circumstances, e.g., worry about possible misfortune to one's child (who is in no danger) and worry about finances (for no good reason), for a period of six months or longer, during which the person has been bothered more days than not by these concerns. In children and adolescents, this may take the form of anxiety and worry about academic, athletic, and social performance.

B. If another Axis I disorder is present, the focus of the anxiety and worry in A is unrelated to it, e.g., the anxiety or worry is not about having a panic attack (as in Panic Disorder), being embarrassed in public (as in Social Phobia), being contaminated (as in Obsessive Compulsive Disorder), or gaining weight (as in Anorexia Nervosa).

C. The disturbance does not occur only during the

course of a Mood Disorder or a psychotic disorder.

D. At least 6 of the following 18 symptoms are often present when anxious (do not include symptoms present only during panic attacks):

Motor tension

(1) trembling, twitching, or feeling shaky
(2) muscle tension, aches, or soreness
(3) restlessness
(4) easy fatigability

Autonomic hyperactivity

(5) shortness of breath or smothering sensations
(6) palpitations or accelerated heart rate (tachycardia)
(7) sweating, or cold clammy hands
(8) dry mouth
(9) dizziness or lightheadedness
(10) nausea, diarrhea, or other abdominal distress
(11) flushes (hot flashes) or chills
(12) frequent urination
(13) trouble swallowing or "lump in throat"

Vigilance and scanning

(14) feeling keyed up or on edge
(15) exaggerated startle response
(16) difficulty concentrating or "mind going blank" because of anxiety
(17) trouble falling or staying asleep
(18) irritability

E. It cannot be established that an organic factor initiated and maintained the disturbance, e.g., hyperthyroidism, Caffeine Intoxication.

300.00 Anxiety Disorder Not Otherwise Specified

Disorders with prominent anxiety or phobic avoidance that are not classifiable as a specific Anxiety Disorder or as an Adjustment Disorder with Anxious Mood.

Somatoform Disorders

300.70 Body Dysmorphic Disorder

A. Preoccupation with some imagined defect in appearance in a normal-appearing person. If a slight physical anomaly is present, the person's concern is grossly excessive.

B. The belief in the defect is not of delusional intensity, as in Delusional Disorder, Somatic Type (i.e, the person can acknowledge the possibility that he or she may be exaggerating the extent of the defect or that there may be no defect at all).

C. Occurrence not exclusively during the course of Anorexia Nervosa or Transsexualism.

300.11 Conversion Disorder (or Hysterical Neurosis, Conversion Type)

A. A loss of, or alteration in, physical functioning suggesting a physical disorder.

B. Psychological factors are judged to be etiologically related to the symptom because of a temporal relationship between a psychosocial stressor that is apparently related to a psychological conflict or need and initiation or exacerbation of the symptom.

C. The person is not conscious of intentionally producing the symptom.

D. The symptom is not a culturally sanctioned response pattern and cannot, after appropriate investigation, be explained by a known physical disorder.

E. The symptom is not limited to pain or to a disturbance in sexual functioning.

Specify: single episode or recurrent.

300.70 Hypochondriasis (or Hypochondriacal Neurosis)

A. Preoccupation with the fear of having, or the belief that one has, a serious disease, based on the person's interpretation of physical signs or sensations as evidence of physical illness.

B. Appropriate physical evaluation does not support the diagnosis of any physical disorder that can account for the physical signs or sensations or the person's unwarranted interpretation of them, **and** the symptoms in A are not just symptoms of panic attacks.

C. The fear of having, or belief that one has, a disease persists despite medical reassurance.

D. Duration of the disturbance is at least six months.

E. The belief in A is not of delusional intensity, as in Delusional Disorder, Somatic Type (i.e, the person can acknowledge the possibility that his or her fear of having, or belief that he or she has, a serious disease is unfounded).

300.81 Somatization Disorder

A. A history of many physical complaints or a belief that one is sickly, beginning before the age of 30 and persisting for several years.

B. At least 13 symptoms from the list below. To count a symptom as significant, the following criteria must be met:

(1) no organic pathology or pathophysiologic mechanism (e.g., a physical disorder or the effects of injury, medication, drugs, or alcohol) to account for the symptom or, when there is related organic pathology, the complaint or resulting social or occupational impairment is grossly in excess of what would be expected from the physical findings

(2) has not occurred only during a panic attack

(3) has caused the person to take medicine (other than over-the-counter pain medication), see a doctor, or alter life-style

Symptom list:

Gastrointestinal symptoms:

(1) **vomiting (other than during pregnancy)**
(2) abdominal pain (other than when menstruating)
(3) nausea (other than motion sickness)
(4) bloating (gassy)
(5) diarrhea
(6) intolerance of (gets sick from) several different foods

Pain symptoms:

(7) **pain in extremities**
(8) back pain

  (9) joint pain
(10) pain during urination
(11) other pain (excluding headaches)

Cardiopulmonary symptoms:

(12) **shortness of breath when not exerting oneself**
(13) palpitations
(14) chest pain
(15) dizziness

Conversion or pseudoneurologic symptoms:

(16) **amnesia**
(17) **difficulty swallowing**
(18) loss of voice
(19) deafness
(20) double vision
(21) blurred vision
(22) blindness
(23) fainting or loss of consciousness
(24) seizure or convulsion
(25) trouble walking
(26) paralysis or muscle weakness
(27) urinary retention or difficulty urinating

Sexual symptoms for the major part of the person's life after opportunities for sexual activity:

(28) **burning sensation in sexual organs or rectum (other than during intercourse)**
(29) sexual indifference
(30) pain during intercourse
(31) impotence

Female reproductive symptoms judged by the person to occur more frequently or severely than in most women:

(32) **painful menstruation**
(33) irregular menstrual periods
(34) excessive menstrual bleeding
(35) vomiting throughout pregnancy

Note: The seven items in boldface may be used to screen for the disorder. The presence of two or more of these items suggests a high likelihood of the disorder.

307.80 Somatoform Pain Disorder

A. Preoccupation with pain for at least six months.

B. Either (1) or (2):

   (1) appropriate evaluation uncovers no organic pathology or pathophysiologic mechanism (e.g., a physical disorder or the effects of injury) to account for the pain

   (2) when there is related organic pathology, the complaint of pain or resulting social or occupational impairment is grossly in excess of what would be expected from the physical findings

300.70 Undifferentiated Somatoform Disorder

A. One or more physical complaints, e.g., fatigue, loss of appetite, gastrointestinal or urinary complaints.

B. Either (1) or (2):

   (1) appropriate evaluation uncovers no organic pathology or pathophysiologic mechanism (e.g., a physical disorder or the effects of injury, medication, drugs, or alcohol) to account for the physical complaints

(2) when there is related organic pathology, the physical complaints or resulting social or occupational impairment is grossly in excess of what would be expected from the physical findings

C. Duration of the disturbance is at least six months.

D. Occurrence not exclusively during the course of another Somatoform Disorder, a Sexual Dysfunction, a Mood Disorder, an Anxiety Disorder, a Sleep Disorder, or a psychotic disorder.

300.70 Somatoform Disorder Not Otherwise Specified

Disorders with somatoform symptoms that do not meet the criteria for any specific Somatoform Disorder or Adjustment Disorder with Physical Complaints.

Examples:

(1) an illness involving nonpsychotic hypochondriacal symptoms of less than six months' duration

(2) an illness involving non-stress-related physical complaints of less than six months' duration.

Dissociative Disorders (or Hysterical Neuroses, Dissociative Type)

300.14 Multiple Personality Disorder

A. The existence within the person of two or more distinct personalities or personality states (each with its own relatively enduring pattern of perceiving, relating to, and thinking about the environment and self).

B. At least two of these personalities or personality states recurrently take full control of the person's behavior.

300.13 Psychogenic Fugue

A. The predominant disturbance is sudden, unexpected travel away from home or one's customary place of work, with inability to recall one's past.

B. Assumption of a new identity (partial or complete).

C. The disturbance is not due to Multiple Personality Disorder or to an Organic Mental Disorder (e.g., partial complex seizures in temporal lobe epilepsy).

300.12 Psychogenic Amnesia

A. The predominant disturbance is an episode of sudden inability to recall important personal information that is too extensive to be explained by ordinary forgetfulness.

B. The disturbance is not due to Multiple Personality Disorder or to an Organic Mental Disorder (e.g., blackouts during Alcohol Intoxication).

300.60 Depersonalization Disorder (or Depersonalization Neurosis)

A. Persistent or recurrent experiences of depersonalization as indicated by either (1) or (2):

   (1) an experience of feeling detached from and as if one is an outside observer of one's mental processes or body
   (2) an experience of feeling like an automaton or as if in a dream

B. During the depersonalization experience, reality testing remains intact.

C. The depersonalization is sufficiently severe and persistent to cause marked distress.

D. The depersonalization experience is the predominant disturbance and is not a symptom of another disorder, such as Schizophrenia, Panic Disorder, or Agoraphobia without History of Panic Disorder but with limited symptom attacks of depersonalization, or temporal lobe epilepsy.

300.15 Dissociative Disorder Not Otherwise Specified

Disorders in which the predominant feature is a dissociative symptom (i.e., a disturbance or alteration in the normally integrative functions of identity, memory, or consciousness) that does not meet the criteria for a specific Dissociative Disorder.

Examples:

(1) Ganser's syndrome: the giving of "approximate answers" to questions, commonly associated with other symptoms, such as amnesia, disorientation, perceptual disturbances, fugue, and conversion symptoms

(2) cases in which there is more than one personality state capable of assuming executive control of the individual, but not more than one personality state is sufficiently distinct to meet the full criteria for Multiple Personality Disorder, or cases in which a second personality never assumes complete executive control

(3) trance states, i.e., altered states of consciousness with markedly diminished or selectively focused responsiveness to environmental stimuli. In children this may occur following physical abuse or trauma.

(4) derealization unaccompanied by depersonalization

(5) dissociated states that may occur in people who have been subjected to periods of prolonged and intense coercive persuasion (e.g., brainwashing, thought reform, or indoctrination while the captive of terrorists or cultists)

(6) cases in which sudden, unexpected travel and organized, purposeful behavior with inability to recall one's past are not accompanied by the assumption of a new identity, partial or complete

Sexual Disorders

PARAPHILIAS

Criteria for severity of manifestations of a specific Paraphilia:

Mild: The person is markedly distressed by the recurrent paraphilic urges, but has never acted on them.

Moderate: The person has occasionally acted on the paraphilic urge.

Severe: The person has repeatedly acted on the paraphilic urge.

302.40 Exhibitionism

A. Over a period of at least six months, recurrent intense sexual urges and sexually arousing fantasies involving the exposure of one's genitals to an unsuspecting stranger.

B. The person has acted on these urges, or is markedly distressed by them.

302.81 Fetishism

A. Over a period of at least six months, recurrent intense sexual urges and sexually arousing fantasies involving the use of nonliving objects by themselves (e.g., female undergarments).

Note: The person may at other times use the non-living object with a sexual partner.

B. The person has acted on these urges, or is markedly distressed by them.

C. The fetishes are not only articles of female clothing used in cross-dressing (Transvestic Fetishism) or devices designed for the purpose of tactile genital stimulation (e.g., vibrator).

302.89 Frotteurism

A. Over a period of at least six months, recurrent intense sexual urges and sexually arousing fantasies involving touching and rubbing against a nonconsenting person. It is the touching, not the coercive nature of the act, that is sexually exciting.

B. The person has acted on these urges, or is markedly distressed by them.

302.20 Pedophilia

A. Over a period of at least six months, recurrent intense sexual urges and sexually arousing fantasies involving sexual activity with a prepubescent child or children (generally age 13 or younger).

B. The person has acted on these urges, or is markedly distressed by them.

C. The person is at least 16 years old and at least 5 years older than the child or children in A.

Note: Do not include a late adolescent involved in an ongoing sexual relationship with a 12- or 13-year-old.

Specify: same sex, opposite sex, or **same and opposite sex.**

Specify if **limited to incest.**

Specify: exclusive type (attracted only to children), or **nonexclusive type.**

302.83 Sexual Masochism

A. Over a period of at least six months, recurrent intense sexual urges and sexually arousing fantasies involving the act (real, not simulated) of being humiliated, beaten, bound, or otherwise made to suffer.

B. The person has acted on these urges, or is markedly distressed by them.

302.84 Sexual Sadism

A. Over a period of at least six months, recurrent intense sexual urges and sexually arousing fantasies involving acts (real, not simulated) in which the psychological or physical suffering (including humiliation) of the victim is sexually exciting to the person.

B. The person has acted on these urges, or is markedly distressed by them.

302.30 Transvestic Fetishism

A. Over a period of at least six months, in a heterosexual male, recurrent intense sexual urges and sexually arousing fantasies involving cross-dressing.

B. The person has acted on these urges, or is markedly distressed by them.

C. Does not meet the criteria for Gender Identity Disorder of Adolescence or Adulthood, Nontranssexual Type, or Transsexualism.

302.82 Voyeurism

A. Over a period of at least six months, recurrent intense sexual urges and sexually arousing fantasies involving the act of observing an unsuspecting person who is naked, in the process of disrobing, or engaging in sexual activity.

B. The person has acted on these urges, or is markedly distressed by them.

302.90 Paraphilia Not Otherwise Specified

Paraphilias that do not meet the criteria for any of the specific categories.

Examples:

(1) Telephone scatologia (lewdness)
(2) Necrophilia (corpses)
(3) Partialism (exclusive focus on part of body)
(4) Zoophilia (animals)
(5) Coprophilia (feces)
(6) Klismaphilia (enemas)
(7) Urophilia (urine)

SEXUAL DYSFUNCTIONS

Specify: psychogenic only, or **psychogenic and biogenic** (Note: If biogenic only, code on Axis III.).

Specify: lifelong or **acquired.**

Specify: generalized or **situational.**

Sexual Desire Disorders

302.71 Hypoactive Sexual Desire Disorder

A. Persistently or recurrently deficient or absent sexual fantasies and desire for sexual activity. The judgment of deficiency or absence is made by the clinician, taking into account factors that affect sexual functioning, such as age, sex, and the context of the person's life.

B. Occurrence not exclusively during the course of another Axis I disorder (other than a Sexual Dysfunction), such as Major Depression.

302.79 Sexual Aversion Disorder

A. Persistent or recurrent extreme aversion to, and avoidance of all, or almost all, genital sexual contact with a sexual partner.

B. Occurrence not exclusively during the course of another Axis I disorder (other than a Sexual Dysfunction), such as Obsessive Compulsive Disorder or Major Depression.

Sexual Arousal Disorders

302.72 Female Sexual Arousal Disorder

A. Either (1) or (2):

   (1) persistent or recurrent partial or complete failure to attain or maintain the lubrication-swelling response of sexual excitement until completion of the sexual activity

   (2) persistent or recurrent lack of a subjective sense of sexual excitement and pleasure in a female during sexual activity

B. Occurrence not exclusively during the course of another Axis I disorder (other than a Sexual Dysfunction), such as Major Depression.

302.72 Male Erectile Disorder

A. Either (1) or (2):
   (1) persistent or recurrent partial or complete failure in a male to attain or maintain erection until completion of the sexual activity
   (2) persistent or recurrent lack of a subjective sense of sexual excitement and pleasure in a male during sexual activity

B. Occurrence not exclusively during the course of another Axis I disorder (other than a Sexual Dysfunction), such as Major Depression.

Orgasm Disorders

302.73 Inhibited Female Orgasm

A. Persistent or recurrent delay in, or absence of, orgasm in a female following a normal sexual excitement phase during sexual activity that the clinician judges to be adequate in focus, intensity, and duration. Some females are able to experience orgasm during noncoital clitoral stimulation, but are unable to experience it during coitus in the absence of manual clitoral stimulation. In most of these females, this represents a normal variation of the female sexual response and does not justify the diagnosis of Inhibited Female Orgasm. However, in some of these females, this does represent a psychological inhibition that justifies the diagnosis. This difficult judgment is assisted by a thorough sexual evaluation, which may even require a trial of treatment.

B. Occurrence not exclusively during the course of another Axis I disorder (other than a Sexual Dysfunction), such as Major Depression.

302.74 Inhibited Male Orgasm

A. Persistent or recurrent delay in, or absence of, orgasm in a male following a normal sexual excitement phase during sexual activity that the clinician, taking into account the person's age, judges to be adequate in focus, intensity, and duration. This failure to achieve orgasm is usually restricted to an inability to reach orgasm in the vagina, with orgasm possible with other types of stimulation, such as masturbation.

B. Occurrence not exclusively during the course of another Axis I disorder (other than a Sexual Dysfunction), such as Major Depression.

302.75 Premature Ejaculation

Persistent or recurrent ejaculation with minimal sexual stimulation or before, upon, or shortly after penetration and before the person wishes it. The clinician must take into account factors that affect duration of the excitement phase, such as age, novelty of the sexual partner or situation, and frequency of sexual activity.

Sexual Pain Disorders

302.76 Dyspareunia

A. Recurrent or persistent genital pain in either a male or a female before, during, or after sexual intercourse.

B. The disturbance is not caused exclusively by lack of lubrication or by Vaginismus.

306.51 Vaginismus

A. Recurrent or persistent involuntary spasm of the musculature of the outer third of the vagina that interferes with coitus.

B. The disturbance is not caused exclusively by a physical disorder, and is not due to another Axis I disorder.

302.70 Sexual Dysfunction Not Otherwise Specified

Sexual Dysfunctions that do not meet the criteria for any of the specific Sexual Dysfunctions.

Examples:

(1) no erotic sensation, or even complete anesthesia, despite normal physiologic components of orgasm
(2) the female analogue of Premature Ejaculation
(3) genital pain during masturbation

OTHER SEXUAL DISORDERS

302.90 Sexual Disorder Not Otherwise Specified

Sexual Disorders that are not classifiable in any of the previous categories. In rare instances, this category may be used concurrently with one of the specific diagnoses when both are necessary to explain or describe the clinical disturbance.

Examples:

(1) marked feelings of inadequacy concerning body habitus, size and shape of sex organs, sexual performance, or other traits related to

self-imposed standards of masculinity or femininity

(2) distress about a pattern of repeated sexual conquests or other forms of nonparaphilic sexual addiction, involving a succession of people who exist only as things to be used

(3) persistent and marked distress about one's sexual orientation

Sleep Disorders

DYSSOMNIAS

Insomnia Disorders

A. The predominant complaint is of difficulty in initiating or maintaining sleep, or of nonrestorative sleep (sleep that is apparently adequate in amount, but leaves the person feeling unrested).

B. The disturbance in A occurs at least three times a week for at least one month and is sufficiently severe to result in either a complaint of significant daytime fatigue or the observation by others of some symptom that is attributable to the sleep disturbance, e.g., irritability or impaired daytime functioning.

C. Occurrence not exclusively during the course of Sleep-Wake Schedule Disorder or a Parasomnia.

307.42 Insomnia Related to Another Mental Disorder (Nonorganic)

Insomnia Disorder, as defined by criteria A, B, and C above, that is related to another Axis I or Axis II mental disorder, such as Major Depression, Generalized Anxiety Disorder, Adjustment Disorder with Anxious Mood, or Obsessive Compulsive Personality Disorder. This category is not used if the Insomnia Disorder is related to an Axis I disorder involving a known organic factor, such as a Psychoactive Substance Use Disorder (e.g., Amphetamine Dependence).

780.50 Insomnia Related to a Known Organic Factor

Insomnia Disorder, as defined by criteria A, B, and C above, that is related to a known organic factor, such as a physical disorder (e.g., sleep apnea, arthritis), a Psychoactive Substance Use Disorder (e.g., Amphetamine Dependence), or a medication (e.g., prolonged use of decongestants).

The known organic factor should be listed on Axis III (if a physical disorder or use of a medication that does not meet the criteria for a Psychoactive Substance Use Disorder) or Axis I (if a Psychoactive Substance Use Disorder).

307.42 Primary Insomnia

Insomnia Disorder, as defined by criteria A, B, and C above, that apparently is not maintained by any other mental disorder or any known organic factor, such as a physical disorder, a Psychoactive Substance Use Disorder, or a medication.

Hypersomnia Disorders

A. The predominant complaint is either (1) or (2):

    (1) excessive daytime sleepiness or sleep attacks not accounted for by an inadequate amount of sleep

    (2) prolonged transition to the fully awake state on awakening (sleep drunkenness)

B. The disturbance in A occurs nearly every day for at least one month, or episodically for longer periods of time, and is sufficiently severe to result in impaired occupational functioning or impairment in usual social activities or relationships with others.

C. Occurrence not exclusively during the course of Sleep-Wake Schedule Disorder.

307.44 Hypersomnia Related to Another Mental Disorder (Nonorganic)

Hypersomnia, as defined by criteria A, B, and C above, that is related to another Axis I or II mental disorder, such as Major Depression or Dysthymia.

780.50 Hypersomnia Related to a Known Organic Factor

Hypersomnia Disorder, as defined by criteria A, B, and C above, that is related to a known organic factor, such as a physical disorder (e.g., sleep apnea), a Psychoactive Substance Use Disorder (e.g., Cannabis Dependence), or a medication (e.g., prolonged use of sedatives or antihypertensives).

The known organic factor should be listed on Axis III (if a physical disorder or use of a medication that does not meet the criteria for a Psychoactive Substance Use Disorder) or Axis I (if a Psychoactive Substance Use Disorder).

780.54 Primary Hypersomnia

Hypersomnia, as defined by criteria A, B, and C above, that is apparently not maintained by any other mental disorder or any known organic factor, such as a physical disorder, a Psychoactive Substance Use Disorder, or a medication.

Sleep-Wake Schedule Disorder

307.45 Sleep-Wake Schedule Disorder

Mismatch between the normal sleep-wake schedule for a person's environment and his or her circadian sleep-wake pattern, resulting in a complaint of either insomnia (criteria A and B of Insomnia Disorder) or hypersomnia (criteria A and B of Hypersomnia Disorder).

Specify type:

Advanced or Delayed Type: Sleep-Wake Schedule Disorder with onset and offset of sleep considerably advanced or delayed (if sleep-wake schedule is not interfered with by medication or environmental demands) in relation to what the person desires (usually the conventional societal sleep-wake schedule).

Disorganized Type: Sleep-Wake Schedule Disorder apparently due to disorganized and variable sleep and waking times, resulting in absence of a daily major sleep period.

Frequently Changing Type: Sleep-Wake Schedule Disorder apparently due to frequently changing sleep and waking times, such as recurrent changes in work shifts or time zones.

Other Dyssomnias

307.40 Dyssomnia Not Otherwise Specified

Insomnias, hypersomnias, or sleep-wake schedule disturbances that cannot be classified in any of the specific categories noted above. An example would be a sleep-wake schedule disturbance apparently related to a physical disorder, such as Parkinson's disease.

PARASOMNIAS

307.47 Dream Anxiety Disorder

A. Repeated awakenings from the major sleep period or naps with detailed recall of extended and extremely frightening dreams, usually involving threats to survival, security, or self-esteem. The awakenings generally occur during the second half of the sleep period.

B. On awakening from the frightening dreams, the person rapidly becomes oriented and alert (in contrast to the confusion and disorientation seen in Sleep Terror Disorder and some forms of epilepsy).

C. The dream experience or the sleep disturbance resulting from the awakenings causes significant distress.

D. It cannot be established that an organic factor initiated and maintained the disturbance, e.g., certain medications.

307.46 Sleep Terror Disorder

A. A predominant disturbance of recurrent episodes of abrupt awakening (lasting 1-10 minutes) from sleep, usually occurring during the first third of the major sleep period and beginning with a panicky scream.

B. Intense anxiety and signs of autonomic arousal during each episode, such as tachycardia, rapid breathing, and sweating, but no detailed dream is recalled.

C. Relative unresponsiveness to efforts of others to comfort the person during the episode and, almost invariably, at least several minutes of confusion, disorientation, and perseverative motor movements (e.g., picking at pillow).

D. It cannot be established that an organic factor initiated and maintained the disturbance, e.g., brain tumor.

307.46 Sleepwalking Disorder

A. Repeated episodes of arising from bed during sleep and walking about, usually occurring during the first third of the major sleep period.

B. While sleepwalking, the person has a blank, staring face, is relatively unresponsive to the efforts of others to influence the sleepwalking or to communicate with him or her, and can be awakened only with great difficulty.

C. On awakening (either from the sleepwalking episode or the next morning), the person has amnesia for the episode.

D. Within several minutes after awakening from the sleepwalking episode, there is no impairment of mental activity or behavior (although there may initially be a short period of confusion or disorientation).

E. It cannot be established that an organic factor initiated and maintained the disturbance, e.g., epilepsy.

307.40 Parasomnia Not Otherwise Specified

Disturbances during sleep that cannot be classified in any of the specified categories noted above. *Example:* Nightmares apparently caused by having taken or withdrawn from certain drugs.

Factitious Disorders

301.51 Factitious Disorder with Physical Symptoms

A. Intentional production or feigning of physical (but not psychological) symptoms.

B. A psychological need to assume the sick role, as evidenced by the absence of external incentives for the behavior, such as economic gain, better care, or physical well-being.

C. Occurrence not exclusively during the course of another Axis I disorder, such as Schizophrenia.

300.16 Factitious Disorder with Psychological Symptoms

A. Intentional production or feigning of psychological (but not physical) symptoms.

B. A psychological need to assume the sick role, as evidenced by the absence of external incentives for the behavior, such as economic gain, better care, or physical well-being.

C. Occurrence not exclusively during the course of another Axis I disorder, such as Schizophrenia.

300.19 Factitious Disorder Not Otherwise Specified

Factitious Disorders that cannot be classified in any of the specific categories, e.g., a disorder with both factitious physical and factitious psychological symptoms.

Impulse Control Disorders Not Elsewhere Classified

312.34 Intermittent Explosive Disorder

A. Several discrete episodes of loss of control of aggressive impulses resulting in serious assaultive acts or destruction of property.

B. The degree of aggressiveness expressed during the episodes is grossly out of proportion to any precipitating psychosocial stressors.

C. There are no signs of generalized impulsiveness or aggressiveness between the episodes.

D. The episodes of loss of control do not occur during the course of a psychotic disorder, Organic Personality Syndrome, Antisocial or Borderline Personality Disorder, Conduct Disorder, or intoxication with a psychoactive substance.

312.32 Kleptomania

A. Recurrent failure to resist impulses to steal objects not needed for personal use or their monetary value.

B. Increasing sense of tension immediately before committing the theft.

C. Pleasure or relief at the time of committing the theft.

D. The stealing is not committed to express anger or vengeance.

E. The stealing is not due to Conduct Disorder or Antisocial Personality Disorder.

312.31 Pathological Gambling

Maladaptive gambling behavior, as indicated by at least four of the following:

(1) frequent preoccupation with gambling or with obtaining money to gamble
(2) frequent gambling of larger amounts of money or over a longer period of time than intended
(3) a need to increase the size or frequency of bets to achieve the desired excitement
(4) restlessness or irritability if unable to gamble
(5) repeated loss of money by gambling and returning another day to win back losses ("chasing")
(6) repeated efforts to reduce or stop gambling
(7) frequent gambling when expected to meet social or occupational obligations
(8) sacrifice of some important social, occupational, or recreational activity in order to gamble
(9) continuation of gambling despite inability to pay mounting debts, or despite other significant social, occupational, or legal problems that the person knows to be exacerbated by gambling

312.33 Pyromania

A. Deliberate and purposeful fire-setting on more than one occasion.

B. Tension or affective arousal before the act.

C. Fascination with, interest in, curiosity about, or attraction to fire and its situational context or associated characteristics (e.g., paraphernalia, uses, consequences, exposure to fires).

D. Intense pleasure, gratification, or relief when setting fires, or when witnessing or participating in their aftermath.

E. The fire-setting is not done for monetary gain, as an expression of sociopolitical ideology, to conceal criminal activity, to express anger or vengeance, to improve one's living circumstances, or in response to a delusion or hallucination.

312.39 Trichotillomania

A. Recurrent failure to resist impulses to pull out one's own hair, resulting in noticeable hair loss.

B. Increasing sense of tension immediately before pulling out the hair.

C. Gratification or a sense of relief when pulling out the hair.

D. No association with a preexisting inflammation of the skin, and not a response to a delusion or hallucination.

312.39 Impulse Control Disorder Not Otherwise Specified

Disorders of impulse control that do not meet the criteria for a specific Impulse Control Disorder.

Adjustment Disorder

A. A reaction to an identifiable psychosocial stressor (or multiple stressors) that occurs within three months of onset of the stressor(s).

B. The maladaptive nature of the reaction is indicated by either of the following:

   (1) impairment in occupational (including school) functioning or in usual social activities or relationships with others
   (2) symptoms that are in excess of a normal and expectable reaction to the stressor(s)

C. The disturbance is not merely one instance of a pattern of overreaction to stress or an exacerbation of one of the mental disorders previously described.

D. The maladaptive reaction has persisted for no longer than six months.

E. The disturbance does not meet the criteria for any specific mental disorder and does not represent Uncomplicated Bereavement.

Types of Adjustment Disorder. Code the type according to the predominant symptoms. Specify the stressor(s) and its (their) severity on Axis IV.

309.24 Adjustment Disorder with Anxious Mood

This category should be used when the predominant manifestation is symptoms such as nervousness, worry, and jitteriness.

309.00 Adjustment Disorder with Depressed Mood

This category should be used when the predominant manifestation is symptoms such as depressed mood, tearfulness, and feelings of hopelessness.

309.30 Adjustment Disorder with Disturbance of Conduct

This category should be used when the predominant manifestation is conduct in which there is violation of the rights of others or of major age-appropriate societal norms and rules. *Examples*: truancy, vandalism, reckless driving, fighting, defaulting on legal responsibilities.

309.40 Adjustment Disorder with Mixed Disturbance of Emotions and Conduct

This category should be used when the predominant manifestations are both emotional symptoms (e.g., depression, anxiety) and a disturbance of conduct (see above).

309.28 Adjustment Disorder with Mixed Emotional Features

This category should be used when the predominant manifestation is a combination of depression and anxiety or other emotions. The major differential is with Depressive and Anxiety Disorders. *Example:* an adolescent who, after moving away from home and parental supervision, reacts with ambivalence, depression, anger, and signs of increased dependence.

309.82 Adjustment Disorder with Physical Complaints

This category should be used when the predominant manifestation is physical symptoms, e.g., fatigue, headache, backache, or other aches and pains, that are not diagnosable as a specific Axis III physical disorder or condition.

309.83 Adjustment Disorder with Withdrawal

This category should be used when the predominant manifestation is social withdrawal without significantly depressed or anxious mood.

309.23 Adjustment Disorder with Work (or Academic) Inhibition

This category should be used when the predominant manifestation is an inhibition in work or academic functioning occurring in a person whose previous work or academic performance has been adequate. Frequently there is also a mixture of anxiety and depression. *Example:* inability to study or to write papers or reports.

309.90 Adjustment Disorder Not Otherwise Specified

Disorders involving maladaptive reactions to psychosocial stressors that are not classifiable as specific types of Adjustment Disorder. *Example:* an immediate reaction to a diagnosis of physical illness, e.g., massive denial and noncompliance, that is too maladaptive to be categorized as the V Code V15.81, Noncompliance with Medical Treatment (p. 206).

Psychological Factors Affecting Physical Condition

316.00 Psychological Factors Affecting Physical Condition

A. Psychologically meaningful environmental stimuli are temporally related to the initiation or exacerbation of a specific physical condition or disorder (recorded on Axis III).

B. The physical condition involves either demonstrable organic pathology (e.g., rheumatoid arthritis) or a known pathophysiologic process (e.g., migraine headache).

C. The condition does not meet the criteria for a Somatoform Disorder.

Personality Disorders

(Note: These are coded on Axis II.)

The diagnostic criteria for the Personality Disorders refer to behaviors or traits that are characteristic of the person's recent (past year) and long-term functioning (generally since adolescence or early adulthood). The constellation of behaviors or traits causes either significant impairment in social or occupational functioning or subjective distress. Behaviors or traits limited to episodes of illness are not considered in making a diagnosis of Personality Disorder.

CLUSTER A

301.00 Paranoid Personality Disorder

A. A pervasive and unwarranted tendency, beginning by early adulthood and present in a variety of contexts, to interpret the actions of people as deliberately demeaning or threatening, as indicated by at least *four* of the following:

   (1) expects, without sufficient basis, to be exploited or harmed by others
   (2) questions, without justification, the loyalty or trustworthiness of friends or associates
   (3) reads hidden demeaning or threatening meanings into benign remarks or events, e.g., sus-

pects that a neighbor put out trash early to annoy him
(4) bears grudges or is unforgiving of insults or slights
(5) is reluctant to confide in others because of unwarranted fear that the information will be used against him or her
(6) is easily slighted and quick to react with anger or to counterattack
(7) questions, without justification, fidelity of spouse or sexual partner

B. Occurrence not exclusively during the course of Schizophrenia or a Delusional Disorder.

301.20 Schizoid Personality Disorder

A. A pervasive pattern of indifference to social relationships and a restricted range of emotional experience and expression, beginning by early adulthood and present in a variety of contexts, as indicated by at least *four* of the following:

(1) neither desires nor enjoys close relationships, including being part of a family
(2) almost always chooses solitary activities
(3) rarely, if ever, claims or appears to experience strong emotions, such as anger and joy
(4) indicates little if any desire to have sexual experiences with another person (age being taken into account)
(5) is indifferent to the praise and criticism of others
(6) has no close friends or confidants (or only one) other than first-degree relatives
(7) displays constricted affect, e.g., is aloof, cold, rarely reciprocates gestures or facial expressions, such as smiles or nods

B. Occurrence not exclusively during the course of Schizophrenia or a Delusional Disorder.

301.22 Schizotypal Personality Disorder

A. A pervasive pattern of deficits in interpersonal relatedness and peculiarities of ideation, appearance, and behavior, beginning by early adulthood and present in a variety of contexts, as indicated by at least *five* of the following:

(1) ideas of reference (excluding delusions of reference)

(2) excessive social anxiety, e.g., extreme discomfort in social situations involving unfamiliar people

(3) odd beliefs or magical thinking, influencing behavior and inconsistent with subcultural norms, e.g., superstitiousness, belief in clairvoyance, telepathy, or "sixth sense," "others can feel my feelings" (in children and adolescents, bizarre fantasies or preoccupations)

(4) unusual perceptual experiences, e.g., illusions, sensing the presence of a force or person not actually present (e.g., "I felt as if my dead mother were in the room with me")

(5) odd or eccentric behavior or appearance, e.g., unkempt, unusual mannerisms, talks to self

(6) no close friends or confidants (or only one) other than first-degree relatives

(7) odd speech (without loosening of associations or incoherence), e.g., speech that is impoverished, digressive, vague, or inappropriately abstract

(8) inappropriate or constricted affect, e.g., silly, aloof, rarely reciprocates gestures or facial expressions, such as smiles or nods

(9) suspiciousness or paranoid ideation

B. Occurrence not exclusively during the course of Schizophrenia or a Pervasive Developmental Disorder.

CLUSTER B

301.70 Antisocial Personality Disorder

A. Current age at least 18.

B. Evidence of Conduct Disorder with onset before age 15, as indicated by a history of *three* or more of the following:

    (1) was often truant

    (2) ran away from home overnight at least twice while living in parental or parental surrogate home (or once without returning)

    (3) often initiated physical fights

    (4) used a weapon in more than one fight

    (5) forced someone into sexual activity with him or her

    (6) was physically cruel to animals

    (7) was physically cruel to other people

    (8) deliberately destroyed others' property (other than by fire-setting)

    (9) deliberately engaged in fire-setting

    (10) often lied (other than to avoid physical or sexual abuse)

    (11) has stolen without confrontation of a victim on more than one occasion (including forgery)

    (12) has stolen with confrontation of a victim (e.g., mugging, purse-snatching, extortion, armed robbery)

C. A pattern of irresponsible and antisocial behavior since the age of 15, as indicated by at least *four* of the following:

(1) is unable to sustain consistent work behavior, as indicated by any of the following (including similar behavior in academic settings if the person is a student):

    (a) significant unemployment for six months or more within five years when expected to work and work was available

    (b) repeated absences from work unexplained by illness in self or family

    (c) abandonment of several jobs without realistic plans for others

(2) fails to conform to social norms with respect to lawful behavior, as indicated by repeatedly performing antisocial acts that are grounds for arrest (whether arrested or not), e.g., destroying property, harassing others, stealing, pursuing an illegal occupation

(3) is irritable and aggressive, as indicated by repeated physical fights or assaults (not required by one's job or to defend someone or oneself), including spouse- or child-beating

(4) repeatedly fails to honor financial obligations, as indicated by defaulting on debts or failing to provide child support or support for other dependents on a regular basis

(5) fails to plan ahead, or is impulsive, as indicated by one or both of the following:

    (a) traveling from place to place without a prearranged job or clear goal for the period of travel or clear idea about when the travel will terminate

    (b) lack of a fixed address for a month or more

(6) has no regard for the truth, as indicated by repeated lying, use of aliases, or "conning" others for personal profit or pleasure

    (7) is reckless regarding his or her own or others' personal safety, as indicated by driving while intoxicated, or recurrent speeding
    (8) if a parent or guardian, lacks ability to function as a responsible parent, as indicated by one or more of the following:

        (a) malnutrition of child
        (b) child's illness resulting from lack of minimal hygiene
        (c) failure to obtain medical care for a seriously ill child
        (d) child's dependence on neighbors or nonresident relatives for food or shelter
        (e) failure to arrange for a caretaker for young child when parent is away from home
        (f) repeated squandering, on personal items, of money required for household necessities

    (9) has never sustained a totally monogamous relationship for more than one year
   (10) lacks remorse (feels justified in having hurt, mistreated, or stolen from another)

D. Occurrence of antisocial behavior not exclusively during the course of Schizophrenia or Manic Episodes.

301.83 Borderline Personality Disorder

A pervasive pattern of instability of mood, interpersonal relationships, and self-image, beginning by early adulthood and present in a variety of contexts, as indicated by at least *five* of the following:

    (1) a pattern of unstable and intense interpersonal relationships characterized by alternating be-

tween extremes of overidealization and de-
valuation

(2) impulsiveness in at least two areas that are
potentially self-damaging, e.g., spending, sex,
substance use, shoplifting, reckless driving,
binge eating (Do not include suicidal or self-
mutilating behavior covered in [5].)

(3) affective instability: marked shifts from base-
line mood to depression, irritability, or anxiety,
usually lasting a few hours and only rarely
more than a few days

(4) inappropriate, intense anger or lack of control
of anger, e.g., frequent displays of temper,
constant anger, recurrent physical fights

(5) recurrent suicidal threats, gestures, or behavior, or self-mutilating behavior

(6) marked and persistent identity disturbance
manifested by uncertainty about at least two of
the following: self-image, sexual orientation,
long-term goals or career choice, type of
friends desired, preferred values

(7) chronic feelings of emptiness or boredom

(8) frantic efforts to avoid real or imagined aban-
donment (Do not include suicidal or self-mutilating behavior covered in [5].)

301.50 Histrionic Personality Disorder

A pervasive pattern of excessive emotionality and at-
tention-seeking, beginning by early adulthood and
present in a variety of contexts, as indicated by at least
four of the following:

(1) constantly seeks or demands reassurance, ap-
proval, or praise

(2) is inappropriately sexually seductive in appearance or behavior

   (3) is overly concerned with physical attractiveness

   (4) expresses emotion with inappropriate exaggeration, e.g., embraces casual acquaintances with excessive ardor, uncontrollable sobbing on minor sentimental occasions, has temper tantrums

   (5) is uncomfortable in situations in which he or she is not the center of attention

   (6) displays rapidly shifting and shallow expression of emotions

   (7) is self-centered, actions being directed toward obtaining immediate satisfaction; has no tolerance for the frustration of delayed gratification

   (8) has a style of speech that is excessively impressionistic and lacking in detail, e.g., when asked to describe mother, can be no more specific than, "She was a beautiful person."

301.81 Narcissistic Personality Disorder

A pervasive pattern of grandiosity (in fantasy or behavior), lack of empathy, and hypersensitivity to the evaluation of others, beginning by early adulthood and present in a variety of contexts, as indicated by at least *five* of the following:

   (1) reacts to criticism with feelings of rage, shame, or humiliation (even if not expressed)

   (2) is interpersonally exploitative: takes advantage of others to achieve his or her own ends

   (3) has a grandiose sense of self-importance, e.g., exaggerates achievements and talents, expects to be noticed as "special" without appropriate achievement

   (4) believes that his or her problems are unique and can be understood only by other special people

(5) is preoccupied with fantasies of unlimited success, power, brilliance, beauty, or ideal love

(6) has a sense of entitlement: unreasonable expectation of especially favorable treatment, e.g., assumes that he or she does not have to wait in line when others must do so

(7) requires constant attention and admiration, e.g., keeps fishing for compliments

(8) lack of empathy: inability to recognize and experience how others feel, e.g., annoyance and surprise when a friend who is seriously ill cancels a date

(9) is preoccupied with feelings of envy

CLUSTER C

301.82 Avoidant Personality Disorder

A pervasive pattern of social discomfort, fear of negative evaluation, and timidity, beginning by early adulthood and present in a variety of contexts, as indicated by at least *four* of the following:

(1) is easily hurt by criticism or disapproval

(2) has no close friends or confidants (or only one) other than first-degree relatives

(3) is unwilling to get involved with people unless certain of being liked

(4) avoids social or occupational activities that involve significant interpersonal contact, e.g., refuses a promotion that will increase social demands

(5) is reticent in social situations because of a fear of saying something inappropriate or foolish, or of being unable to answer a question

(6) fears being embarrassed by blushing, crying, or showing signs of anxiety in front of other people

(7) exaggerates the potential difficulties, physical dangers, or risks involved in doing something ordinary but outside his or her usual routine, e.g., may cancel social plans because she anticipates being exhausted by the effort of getting there

301.60 Dependent Personality Disorder

A pervasive pattern of dependent and submissive behavior, beginning by early adulthood and present in a variety of contexts, as indicated by at least *five* of the following:

(1) is unable to make everyday decisions without an excessive amount of advice or reassurance from others
(2) allows others to make most of his or her important decisions, e.g., where to live, what job to take
(3) agrees with people even when he or she believes they are wrong, because of fear of being rejected
(4) has difficulty initiating projects or doing things on his or her own
(5) volunteers to do things that are unpleasant or demeaning in order to get other people to like him or her
(6) feels uncomfortable or helpless when alone, or goes to great lengths to avoid being alone
(7) feels devastated or helpless when close relationships end
(8) is frequently preoccupied with fears of being abandoned
(9) is easily hurt by criticism or disapproval

301.40 Obsessive Compulsive Personality Disorder

A pervasive pattern of perfectionism and inflexibility, beginning by early adulthood and present in a variety of contexts, as indicated by at least *five* of the following:

(1) perfectionism that interferes with task completion, e.g., inability to complete a project because own overly strict standards are not met

(2) preoccupation with details, rules, lists, order, organization, or schedules to the extent that the major point of the activity is lost

(3) unreasonable insistence that others submit to exactly his or her way of doing things, **or** unreasonable reluctance to allow others to do things because of the conviction that they will not do them correctly

(4) excessive devotion to work and productivity to the exclusion of leisure activities and friendships (not accounted for by obvious economic necessity)

(5) indecisiveness: decision making is either avoided, postponed, or protracted, e.g., the person cannot get assignments done on time because of ruminating about priorities (do not include if indecisiveness is due to excessive need for advice or reassurance from others)

(6) overconscientiousness, scrupulousness, and inflexibility about matters of morality, ethics, or values (not accounted for by cultural or religious identification)

(7) restricted expression of affection

(8) lack of generosity in giving time, money, or gifts when no personal gain is likely to result

(9) inability to discard worn-out or worthless ob-

jects even when they have no sentimental value

301.84 Passive Aggressive Personality Disorder

A pervasive pattern of passive resistance to demands for adequate social and occupational performance, beginning by early adulthood and present in a variety of contexts, as indicated by at least *five* of the following:

(1) procrastinates, i.e., puts off things that need to be done so that deadlines are not met
(2) becomes sulky, irritable, or argumentative when asked to do something he or she does not want to do
(3) seems to work deliberately slowly or to do a bad job on tasks that he or she really does not want to do
(4) protests, without justification, that others make unreasonable demands on him or her
(5) avoids obligations by claiming to have "forgotten"
(6) believes that he or she is doing a much better job than others think he or she is doing
(7) resents useful suggestions from others concerning how he or she could be more productive
(8) obstructs the efforts of others by failing to do his or her share of the work
(9) unreasonably criticizes or scorns people in positions of authority

301.90 Personality Disorder Not Otherwise Specified

Disorders of personality functioning that are not classifiable as a specific Personality Disorder. An example is features of more than one specific Personality Disorder that do not meet the full criteria for any one disorder, yet cause significant impairment in social or occupational functioning, or subjective distress. In DSM-III, this was called Mixed Personality Disorder.

This category can also be used when the clinician judges that a specific Personality Disorder not included in this classification is appropriate, such as Impulsive Personality Disorder, Immature Personality Disorder, Self-defeating Personality Disorder (see p. 216), or Sadistic Personality Disorder (see p. 214). In such instances the clinician should note the specific personality disorder in parentheses, e.g., Personality Disorder NOS (Self-defeating Personality Disorder).

V Codes for Conditions Not Attributable to a Mental Disorder That Are a Focus of Attention or Treatment

The ICD-9-CM includes V Codes for a "Supplementary Classification of Factors Influencing Health Status and Contact with Health Services." A brief list of V Codes adapted from ICD-9-CM is provided here for conditions that are a focus of attention or treatment but are not attributable to any of the mental disorders noted previously. In some instances, a thorough evaluation has failed to uncover any mental disorder; in other instances, the scope of the diagnostic evaluation has not been adequate to determine the presence or absence of a mental disorder, but there is a need to note the reason for contact with the mental health care system. (With further information, the presence of a mental disorder may become apparent.) Finally, a person may have a mental disorder, but the focus of attention or treatment may be on a condition that is not due to the mental disorder. For example, a person with Bipolar Disorder may have marital problems that are not directly related to manifestations of the Mood Disorder but are the principal focus of treatment.

V62.30 Academic Problem

This category can be used when the focus of attention or treatment is an academic problem that is apparently not due to a mental disorder. An example is a pattern of failing grades or of significant under-achievement in a person with adequate intellectual capacity in the absence of a Specific Developmental Disorder or any other mental disorder that would account for the problem.

V71.01 Adult Antisocial Behavior

This category can be used when the focus of attention or treatment is adult antisocial behavior that is apparently not due to a mental disorder, such as Conduct Disorder, Antisocial Personality Disorder, or an Impulse Control Disorder. Examples include the behavior of some professional thieves, racketeers, or dealers in illegal psychoactive substances.

V40.00 Borderline Intellectual Functioning
Note: This is coded on Axis II.

This category can be used when the focus of attention or treatment is associated with Borderline Intellectual Functioning, i.e., an IQ in the 71–84 range. Differential diagnosis between Borderline Intellectual Functioning and Mental Retardation (an IQ of 70 or below) is especially difficult and important when the coexistence of certain mental disorders is involved. For example, when the diagnosis is Schizophrenia, Undifferentiated or Residual Type, and impairment in adaptive functioning is prominent, the existence of Borderline Intellectual Functioning is easily overlooked, and hence the level and quality of potentially adaptive functioning may be incorrectly assessed.

V71.02 Childhood or Adolescent Antisocial Behavior

This category can be used when the focus of attention or treatment is antisocial behavior in a child or adolescent that is apparently not due to a mental disorder, such as Conduct Disorder, Antisocial Personality Disorder, or an Impulse Control Disorder. Examples include isolated antisocial acts of children or adolescents (not a pattern of antisocial behavior).

V65.20 Malingering

The essential feature of Malingering is intentional production of false or grossly exaggerated physical or psychological symptoms, motivated by external incentives such as avoiding military conscription or duty, avoiding work, obtaining financial compensation, evading criminal prosecution, obtaining drugs, or securing better living conditions.

Under some circumstances Malingering may represent adaptive behavior, for example, feigning illness while a captive of the enemy during wartime.

Malingering should be strongly suspected if any combination of the following is noted:

(1) medicolegal context of presentation, e.g., the person's being referred by his or her attorney to the physician for examination;

(2) marked discrepancy between the person's claimed stress or disability and the objective findings;

(3) lack of cooperation during the diagnostic evaluation and in complying with the prescribed treatment regimen;

(4) the presence of Antisocial Personality Disorder.

Malingering differs from Factitious Disorder in that the motivation for the symptom production in Malingering is external incentives, whereas in Factitious Disorder there is an absence of external incentives. Evidence of an intrapsychic need to maintain the sick role suggests Factitious Disorder. Thus, a diagnosis of Factitious Disorder excludes a diagnosis of Malingering.

Malingering is differentiated from Conversion and other Somatoform Disorders by the intentional production of symptoms and by the obvious, external incentives. The person who is malingering is much less likely to present his or her symptoms in the context of emotional conflict, and the presenting symptoms are less likely to be symbolically related to an underlying emotional conflict. Symptom relief in Malingering is not often obtained by suggestion, hypnosis, or an amobarbital interview, as it frequently is in Conversion Disorder.

V61.10 Marital Problem

This category can be used when the focus of attention or treatment is a marital problem that is apparently not due to a mental disorder. An example is marital conflict related to estrangement or divorce.

V15.81 Noncompliance with Medical Treatment

This category can be used when the focus of attention or treatment is noncompliance with medical treatment that is apparently not due to a mental disorder. Examples include: irrationally motivated noncompliance due to denial of illness, noncompliance due to religious beliefs, and decisions based on personal value judgments about the advantages and disadvantages of the proposed treatment. The category should not be used if the noncompliance is due to a mental disorder, such as Schizophrenia or a Psychoactive Substance Use Disorder.

V62.20 Occupational Problem

This category can be used when the focus of attention or treatment is an occupational problem that is apparently not due to a mental disorder. Examples include job dissatisfaction and uncertainty about career choices.

V61.20 Parent–Child Problem

This category can be used for either a parent or a child when the focus of attention or treatment is a parent–child problem that is apparently not due to a mental disorder of the person who is being evaluated. An example is conflict between a mentally healthy adolescent and her parents about her choice of friends.

V62.81 Other Interpersonal Problem

This category can be used when the focus of attention or treatment is an interpersonal problem (other than marital or parent–child) that is apparently not due to a mental disorder of the person who is being evaluated. Examples are difficulties with co-workers, or with romantic partners.

V61.80 Other Specified Family Circumstances

This category can be used when the focus of attention or treatment is a family circumstance that is apparently not due to a mental disorder and is not a Parent–Child or a Marital Problem. Examples are interpersonal difficulties with an aged in-law, or sibling rivalry.

V62.89 Phase of Life Problem or Other Life Circumstance Problem

This category can be used when the focus of attention or treatment is a problem associated with a particular developmental phase or some other life circumstance that is apparently not due to a mental disorder. Examples include problems associated with entering school, leaving parental control, starting a new career, and changes involved in marriage, divorce, and retirement.

V62.82 Uncomplicated Bereavement

This category can be used when the focus of attention or treatment is a normal reaction to the death of a loved one (bereavement).

A full depressive syndrome frequently is a normal reaction to such a loss, with feelings of depression and such associated symptoms as poor appetite, weight loss, and insomnia. However, morbid preoccupation with worthlessness, prolonged and marked functional impairment, and marked psychomotor retardation are uncommon and suggest that the bereavement is complicated by the development of a Major Depression.

In Uncomplicated Bereavement, guilt, if present, is chiefly about things done or not done by the survivor at the time of the death; thoughts of death are usually limited to the person's thinking that he or she would be better off dead or that he or she should have died with the deceased person. The person with Uncomplicated Bereavement generally regards the feeling of depressed mood as "normal," although he or she may seek professional help for relief of such associated symptoms as insomnia or anorexia.

The reaction to the loss may not be immediate, but rarely occurs after the first two or three months. The duration of "normal" bereavement varies considerably among different cultural groups.

Additional Codes

Note: Although the terms below distinguish between Axis I and Axis II, in order to maintain compatibility with ICD-9-CM, these Axis I and Axis II codes are the same.

300.90 Unspecified Mental Disorder (Nonpsychotic)

When enough information is available to rule out a psychotic disorder, but further specification is not possible, the residual category Unspecified Mental Disorder (Nonpsychotic) is used. In some cases, with more information the diagnosis can be changed to a specific disorder. This category can also be used for specific mental disorders that are not included in the DSM-III-R classification, for example, Late Luteal Phase Dysphoric Disorder.

V71.09 No Diagnosis or Condition on Axis I

When no Axis I diagnosis or condition (including the V code categories) is present, this should be indicated. There may or may not be an Axis II diagnosis.

799.90 Diagnosis or Condition Deferred on Axis I

When there is insufficient information to make any diagnostic judgment about an Axis I diagnosis or condition, this should be noted as Diagnosis or Condition Deferred on Axis I.

V71.09 No Diagnosis on Axis II

When no Axis II diagnosis (i.e., no Personality Disorder or Specific Developmental Disorder) is present, this should be indicated. There may or may not be an Axis I diagnosis or condition.

799.90 Diagnosis Deferred on Axis II

When there is insufficient information to make any diagnostic judgment about an Axis II diagnosis, this should be noted as Diagnosis Deferred on Axis II.

Proposed Diagnostic Categories Needing Further Study

Proposed Diagnostic Categories Needing Further Study

This appendix presents three diagnoses that were proposed for inclusion in DSM-III-R. They are included here to facilitate further systematic clinical study and research.

Diagnostic criteria for Late Luteal Phase Dysphoric Disorder

A. In most menstrual cycles during the past year, symptoms in B occurred during the last week of the luteal phase and remitted within a few days after onset of the follicular phase. In menstruating females, these phases correspond to the week before, and a few days after, the onset of menses. (In nonmenstruating females who have had a hysterectomy, the timing of luteal and follicular phases may require measurement of circulating reproductive hormones.)

B. At least five of the following symptoms have been present for most of the time during each symptomatic late luteal phase, at least one of the symptoms being either (1), (2), (3), or (4):

   (1) marked affective lability, e.g., feeling suddenly sad, tearful, irritable, or angry
   (2) persistent and marked anger or irritability
   (3) marked anxiety, tension, feelings of being "keyed up" or "on edge"

(4) markedly depressed mood, feelings of hopelessness, or self-deprecating thoughts

(5) decreased interest in usual activities, e.g., work, friends, hobbies

(6) easy fatigability or marked lack of energy

(7) subjective sense of difficulty in concentrating

(8) marked change in appetite, overeating, or specific food cravings

(9) hypersomnia or insomnia

(10) other physical symptoms, such as breast tenderness or swelling, headaches, joint or muscle pain, a sensation of "bloating," weight gain

C. The disturbance seriously interferes with work or with usual social activities or relationships with others.

D. The disturbance is not merely an exacerbation of the symptoms of another disorder, such as Major Depression, Panic Disorder, Dysthymia, or a Personality Disorder (although it may be superimposed on any of these disorders).

E. Criteria A, B, C, and D are confirmed by prospective daily self-ratings during at least two symptomatic cycles. (The diagnosis may be made provisionally prior to this confirmation.)

Note: For coding purposes, record: 300.90 Unspecified Mental Disorder (Late Luteal Phase Dysphoric Disorder).

Diagnostic criteria for Sadistic Personality Disorder

A. A pervasive pattern of cruel, demeaning, and aggressive behavior, beginning by early adulthood, as indicated by the repeated occurrence of at least four of the following:

(1) has used physical cruelty or violence for the purpose of establishing dominance in a relationship (not merely to achieve some noninterpersonal goal, such as striking someone in order to rob him or her)

(2) humiliates or demeans people in the presence of others

(3) has treated or disciplined someone under his or her control unusually harshly, e.g., a child, student, prisoner, or patient

(4) is amused by, or takes pleasure in, the psychological or physical suffering of others (including animals)

(5) has lied for the purpose of harming or inflicting pain on others (not merely to achieve some other goal)

(6) gets other people to do what he or she wants by frightening them (through intimidation or even terror)

(7) restricts the autonomy of people with whom he or she has a close relationship, e.g., will not let spouse leave the house unaccompanied or permit teen-age daughter to attend social functions

(8) is fascinated by violence, weapons, martial arts, injury, or torture

B. The behavior in A has not been directed toward only one person (e.g., spouse, one child) and has not been solely for the purpose of sexual arousal (as in Sexual Sadism).

Note: For coding purposes, record: 301.90 Personality Disorder NOS (Sadistic Personality Disorder).

Diagnostic criteria for Self-defeating Personality Disorder

A. A pervasive pattern of self-defeating behavior, beginning by early adulthood and present in a variety of contexts. The person may often avoid or undermine pleasurable experiences, be drawn to situations or relationships in which he or she will suffer, and prevent others from helping him or her, as indicated by at least five of the following:

   (1) chooses people and situations that lead to disappointment, failure, or mistreatment even when better options are clearly available

   (2) rejects or renders ineffective the attempts of others to help him or her

   (3) following positive personal events (e.g., new achievement), responds with depression, guilt, or a behavior that produces pain (e.g., an accident)

   (4) incites angry or rejecting responses from others and then feels hurt, defeated, or humiliated (e.g., makes fun of spouse in public, provoking an angry retort, then feels devastated)

   (5) rejects opportunities for pleasure, or is reluctant to acknowledge enjoying himself or herself (despite having adequate social skills and the capacity for pleasure)

   (6) fails to accomplish tasks crucial to his or her personal objectives despite demonstrated ability to do so, e.g., helps fellow students write papers, but is unable to write his or her own

   (7) is uninterested in or rejects people who consistently treat him or her well, e.g., is unattracted to caring sexual partners

   (8) engages in excessive self-sacrifice that is un-

      solicited by the intended recipients of the sacrifice

B. The behaviors in A do not occur exclusively in response to, or in anticipation of, being physically, sexually, or psychologically abused.

C. The behaviors in A do not occur only when the person is depressed.

Note: For coding purposes, record: 301.90 Personality Disorder NOS (Self-defeating Personality Disorder).

Decision Trees for
Differential Diagnosis

The purpose of these decision trees is to aid the clinician in understanding the organization and hierarchic structure of the classification. Each decision tree starts with a set of clinical features. When one of these features is a prominent part of the presenting clinical picture, either as current or past symptomatology, the clinician can follow the series of questions to rule in or out various disorders. Since the classification may allow several disorders to be diagnosed within a diagnostic area (for example, Social Phobia and Obsessive Compulsive Disorder in Anxiety Disorders), the clinician should proceed down the tree until a leaf (i.e., a point in the tree with no outgoing branches) is found. If features from several different trees are present, each of the appropriate trees should be examined. For example, if a mood disturbance and psychotic symptoms are *both* present, both the MOOD and the PSYCHOTIC trees should be explored.

Note: Many of the questions only approximate the actual criteria.

Decision Trees for Differential Diagnosis[1]

I.	Psychotic symptoms	p. 222
II.	Mood disturbance	p. 224
III.	Specific organic factor likely	p. 226
IV.	Irrational anxiety, avoidance behavior, and increased arousal	p. 228
V.	Physical complaints or anxiety about illness	p. 230

---

[1] Prepared by Michael B. First, M.D., Janet B.W. Williams, D.S.W., and Robert L. Spitzer, M.D.

Differential Diagnosis of Psychotic Symptoms

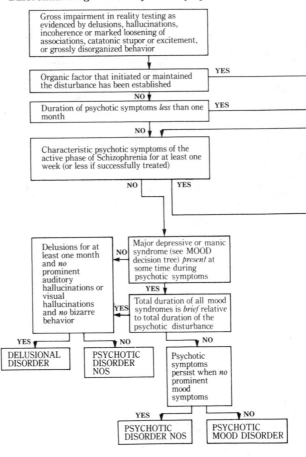

→ See ORGANIC decision tree

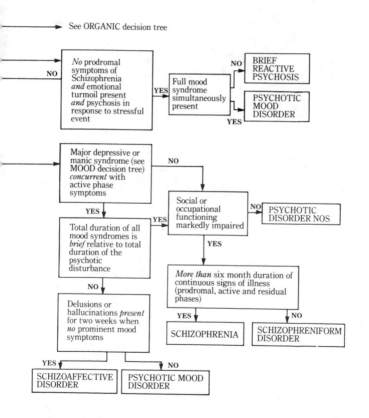

Differential Diagnosis of Mood Disturbances

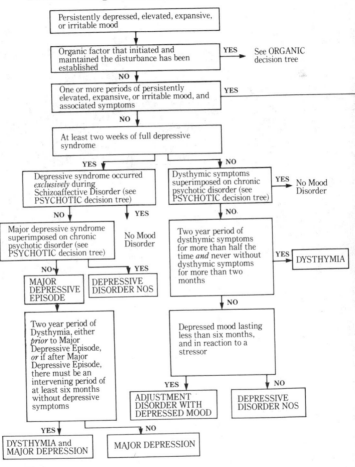

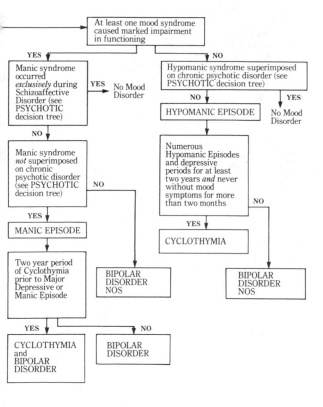

Differential Diagnosis of Organic Mental Disorders

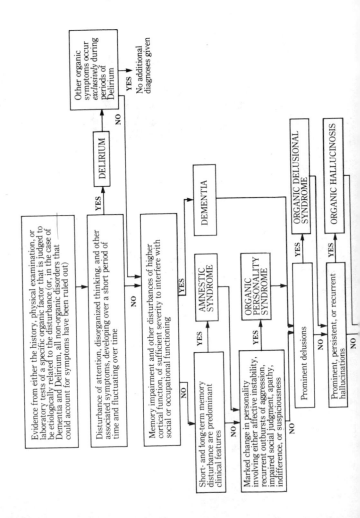

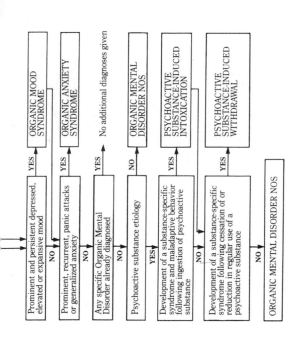

Prominent and persistent depressed, elevated or expansive mood	YES →	ORGANIC MOOD SYNDROME
↓ NO		
Prominent, recurrent, panic attacks or generalized anxiety	YES →	ORGANIC ANXIETY SYNDROME
↓ NO		
Any specific Organic Mental Disorder already diagnosed	YES →	No additional diagnoses given
↓ NO		
Psychoactive substance etiology	NO →	ORGANIC MENTAL DISORDER NOS
↓ YES		
Development of a substance-specific syndrome and maladaptive behavior following ingestion of psychoactive substance	YES →	PSYCHOACTIVE SUBSTANCE-INDUCED INTOXICATION
↓ NO		
Development of a substance-specific syndrome following cessation of or reduction in regular use of a psychoactive substance	YES →	PSYCHOACTIVE SUBSTANCE-INDUCED WITHDRAWAL
↓ NO		
ORGANIC MENTAL DISORDER NOS		

Differential Diagnosis of Anxiety Disorders

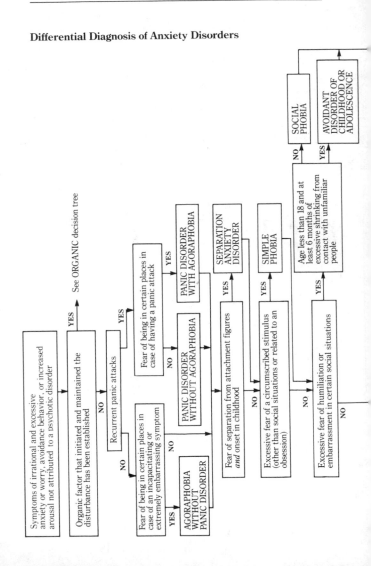

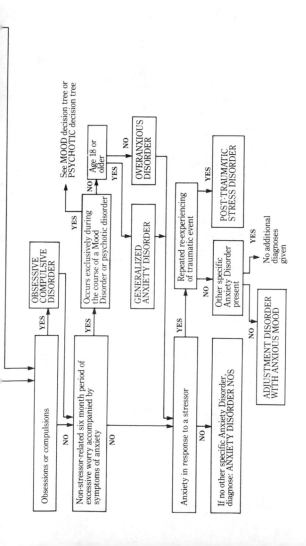

Differential Diagnosis of Somatoform Disorders

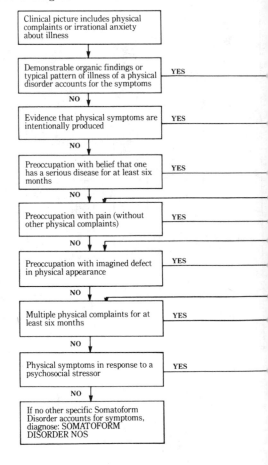

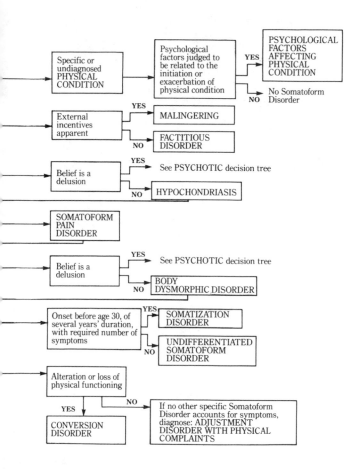

Alphabetic Listing
of DSM-III-R Diagnoses

Alphabetic Listing
of DSM-III-R Diagnoses

V62.30	Academic problem
309.90	Adjustment disorder NOS
	Adjustment disorder
309.24	with anxious mood
309.00	with depressed mood
309.30	with disturbance of conduct
309.40	with mixed disturbance of emotions and conduct
309.28	with mixed emotional features
309.82	with physical complaints
309.83	with withdrawal
309.23	with work (or academic) inhibition
V71.01	Adult antisocial behavior
300.22	Agoraphobia without history of panic disorder
	Alcohol
305.00	abuse
291.10	amnestic disorder
303.90	dependence
291.30	hallucinosis
291.40	idiosyncratic intoxication
303.00	intoxication
291.00	withdrawal delirium
294.00	Amnestic disorder (etiology noted on Axis III or is unknown)

	Amphetamine or similarly acting sympathomimetic
305.70	abuse
292.81	delirium
292.11	delusional disorder
304.40	dependence
305.70	intoxication
292.00	withdrawal
307.10	Anorexia nervosa
301.70	Antisocial personality disorder
300.00	Anxiety disorder NOS
314.01	Attention-deficit hyperactivity disorder
299.00	Autistic disorder
313.21	Avoidant disorder of childhood or adolescence
301.82	Avoidant personality disorder
296.70	Bipolar disorder NOS
	Bipolar disorder, depressed,
296.56	in full remission
296.55	in partial remission
296.51	mild
296.52	moderate
296.53	severe, without psychotic features
296.50	unspecified
296.54	with psychotic features
	Bipolar disorder, manic,
296.46	in full remission
296.45	in partial remission
296.41	mild
296.42	moderate
296.43	severe, without psychotic features
296.40	unspecified
296.44	with psychotic features
	Bipolar disorder, mixed,
296.66	in full remission
296.65	in partial remission
296.61	mild
296.62	moderate

296.63	severe, without psychotic features
296.60	unspecified
296.64	with psychotic features
300.70	Body dysmorphic disorder
V40.00	Borderline intellectual functioning
301.83	Borderline personality disorder
298.80	Brief reactive psychosis
307.51	Bulimia nervosa
305.90	Caffeine intoxication
	Cannabis
305.20	abuse
292.11	delusional disorder
304.30	dependence
305.20	intoxication
V71.02	Childhood or adolescent antisocial behavior
307.22	Chronic motor or vocal tic disorder
307.00	Cluttering
	Cocaine
305.60	abuse
292.81	delirium
292.11	delusional disorder
304.20	dependence
305.60	intoxication
292.00	withdrawal
	Conduct disorder,
312.20	group type
312.00	solitary aggressive type
312.90	undifferentiated type
300.11	Conversion disorder
301.13	Cyclothymia
293.00	Delirium (etiology noted on Axis III or is unknown)
297.10	Delusional disorder
294.10	Dementia (etiology noted on Axis III or is unknown)
291.20	Dementia associated with alcoholism
301.60	Dependent personality disorder

300.60	Depersonalization disorder
311.00	Depressive disorder NOS
	Developmental
315.10	arithmetic disorder
315.39	articulation disorder
315.40	coordination disorder
315.90	disorder NOS
315.31	expressive language disorder
315.80	expressive writing disorder
315.00	reading disorder
315.31	receptive language disorder
799.90	Diagnosis or condition deferred on Axis I
799.90	Diagnosis or condition deferred on Axis II
300.15	Dissociative disorder NOS
307.47	Dream anxiety disorder (Nightmare disorder)
302.76	Dyspareunia
307.40	Dyssomnia NOS
300.40	Dysthymia
307.50	Eating Disorder NOS
313.23	Elective mutism
302.40	Exhibitionism
300.19	Factitious disorder NOS
	Factitious disorder
301.51	with physical symptoms
300.16	with psychological symptoms
302.72	Female sexual arousal disorder
302.81	Fetishism
302.89	Frotteurism
307.70	Functional encopresis
307.60	Functional enuresis
	Gender identity disorder
302.85	NOS
302.85	of adolescence or adulthood, nontranssexual type
302.60	of childhood
300.02	Generalized anxiety disorder

	Hallucinogen
305.30	abuse
292.11	delusional disorder
304.50	dependence
305.30	hallucinosis
292.84	mood disorder
301.50	Histrionic personality disorder
780.50	Hypersomnia related to a known organic factor
307.44	Hypersomnia related to another mental disorder (nonorganic)
302.71	Hypoactive sexual desire disorder
300.70	Hypochondriasis
313.82	Identity disorder
312.39	Impulse control disorder NOS
297.30	Induced psychotic disorder
	Inhalant
305.90	abuse
304.60	dependence
305.90	intoxication
302.73	Inhibited female orgasm
302.74	Inhibited male orgasm
780.50	Insomnia related to a known organic factor
307.42	Insomnia related to another mental disorder (nonorganic)
312.34	Intermittent explosive disorder
312.32	Kleptomania
307.90	Late luteal phase dysphoric disorder
	Major depression, recurrent,
296.36	in full remission
296.35	in partial remission
296.31	mild
296.32	moderate
296.33	severe, without psychotic features
296.30	unspecified
296.34	with psychotic features

	Major depression, single episode,
296.26	in full remission
296.25	in partial remission
296.21	mild
296.22	moderate
296.23	severe, without psychotic features
296.20	unspecified
296.24	with psychotic features
302.72	Male erectile disorder
V65.20	Malingering
V61.10	Marital problem
317.00	Mild mental retardation
318.00	Moderate mental retardation
	Multi-infarct dementia,
290.40	uncomplicated
290.41	with delirium
290.42	with delusions
290.43	with depression
300.14	Multiple personality disorder
301.81	Narcissistic personality disorder
	Nicotine
305.10	dependence
292.00	withdrawal
V71.09	No diagnosis or condition on Axis I
V71.09	No diagnosis or condition on Axis II
V15.81	Noncompliance with medical treatment
300.30	Obsessive compulsive disorder
301.40	Obsessive compulsive personality disorder
V62.20	Occupational problem
	Opioid
305.50	abuse
304.00	dependence
305.50	intoxication
292.00	withdrawal
313.81	Oppositional defiant disorder
294.80	Organic anxiety disorder (etiology noted on Axis III or is unknown)

293.81	Organic delusional disorder (etiology noted on Axis III or is unknown)
293.82	Organic hallucinosis (etiology noted on Axis III or is unknown)
294.80	Organic mental disorder NOS (etiology noted on Axis III or is unknown)
293.83	Organic mood disorder (etiology noted on Axis III or is unknown)
310.10	Organic personality disorder (etiology noted on Axis III or is unknown)
	Other or unspecified psychoactive substance
292.83	amnestic disorder
292.89	anxiety disorder
292.81	delirium
292.11	delusional disorder
292.82	dementia
292.12	hallucinosis
305.90	intoxication
292.84	mood disorder
292.90	organic mental disorder NOS
292.89	personality disorder
292.00	withdrawal
V62.81	Other interpersonal problem
V61.80	Other specified family circumstances
313.00	Overanxious disorder
	Panic disorder
300.21	with agoraphobia
300.01	without agoraphobia
301.00	Paranoid personality disorder
302.90	Paraphilia NOS
307.40	Parasomnia NOS
V61.20	Parent-child problem
301.84	Passive aggressive personality disorder
312.31	Pathological gambling
302.20	Pedophilia
301.90	Personality disorder NOS

299.80	Pervasive developmental disorder NOS
V62.89	Phase of life problem or other life circumstance problem
	Phencyclidine (PCP) or similarly acting arylcyclohexylamine
305.90	abuse
292.81	delirium
292.11	delusional disorder
304.50	dependence
305.90	intoxication
292.84	mood disorder
292.90	organic mental disorder NOS
307.52	Pica
305.90	Polysubstance abuse
304.90	Polysubstance dependence
292.89	Posthallucinogen perception disorder
309.89	Post-traumatic stress disorder
302.75	Premature ejaculation
290.10	Presenile dementia NOS
	Primary degenerative dementia of the Alzheimer type,
290.11	presenile onset, with delirium
290.12	presenile onset, with delusions
290.13	presenile onset, with depression
290.10	presenile onset, uncomplicated
	Primary degenerative dementia of the Alzheimer type,
290.30	senile onset, with delirium
290.20	senile onset, with delusions
290.21	senile onset, with depression
290.00	senile onset, uncomplicated
780.54	Primary hypersomnia
307.42	Primary insomnia
318.20	Profound mental retardation
305.90	Psychoactive substance abuse NOS
304.90	Psychoactive substance dependence NOS
300.12	Psychogenic amnesia

300.13	Psychogenic fugue
316.00	Psychological factors affecting physical condition
298.90	Psychotic disorder NOS
312.33	Pyromania
313.89	Reactive attachment disorder of infancy or early childhood
307.53	Rumination disorder of infancy
295.70	Schizoaffective disorder
301.20	Schizoid personality disorder
	Schizophrenia, catatonic type,
295.22	chronic
295.24	chronic with acute exacerbation
295.21	subchronic
295.23	subchronic with acute exacerbation
295.20	unspecified
	Schizophrenia, disorganized type,
295.12	chronic
295.14	chronic with acute exacerbation
295.11	subchronic
295.13	subchronic with acute exacerbation
295.10	unspecified
	Schizophrenia, paranoid type,
295.32	chronic
295.34	chronic with acute exacerbation
295.31	subchronic
295.33	subchronic with acute exacerbation
295.30	unspecified
	Schizophrenia, residual type,
295.62	chronic
295.64	chronic with acute exacerbation
295.61	subchronic
295.63	subchronic with acute exacerbation
295.60	unspecified
	Schizophrenia, undifferentiated type,
295.92	chronic
295.94	chronic with acute exacerbation

295.91	subchronic
295.93	subchronic with acute exacerbation
295.95	unspecified
295.40	Schizophreniform disorder
301.22	Schizotypal personality disorder
	Sedative, hypnotic, or anxiolytic
305.40	abuse
292.83	amnestic disorder
304.10	dependence
305.40	intoxication
292.00	withdrawal delirium
290.00	Senile dementia NOS
309.21	Separation anxiety disorder
318.10	Severe mental retardation
302.79	Sexual aversion disorder
302.90	Sexual disorder NOS
302.70	Sexual dysfunction NOS
302.83	Sexual masochism
302.84	Sexual sadism
300.29	Simple phobia
307.46	Sleep terror disorder
307.45	Sleep-wake schedule disorder
307.46	Sleepwalking disorder
300.23	Social phobia
300.81	Somatization disorder
300.70	Somatoform disorder NOS
307.80	Somatoform pain disorder
315.90	Specific developmental disorder NOS
307.30	Stereotypy/habit disorder
307.00	Stuttering
307.20	Tic disorder NOS
307.23	Tourette's disorder
307.21	Transient tic disorder
302.50	Transsexualism
302.30	Transvestic fetishism
312.39	Trichotillomania
291.80	Uncomplicated alcohol withdrawal

V62.82	Uncomplicated bereavement
292.00	Uncomplicated sedative, hypnotic, or anxiolytic withdrawal
314.00	Undifferentiated attention-deficit disorder
300.70	Undifferentiated somatoform disorder
300.90	Unspecified mental disorder (nonpsychotic)
319.00	Unspecified mental retardation
306.51	Vaginismus
302.82	Voyeurism

Numeric Listing
of DSM-III-R Codes

In order to maintain compatibility with ICD-9-CM, some DSM-III-R diagnoses share the same code numbers. These are indicated in this list by a bracket.

290.00	Primary degenerative dementia of the Alzheimer type, senile onset, uncomplicated
290.00	Senile dementia NOS
290.10	Presenile dementia NOS
290.10	Primary degenerative dementia of the Alzheimer type, presenile onset, uncomplicated
290.11	Primary degenerative dementia of the Alzheimer type, presenile onset, with delirium
290.12	Primary degenerative dementia of the Alzheimer type, presenile onset, with delusions
290.13	Primary degenerative dementia of the Alzheimer type, presenile onset, with depression
290.20	Primary degenerative dementia of the Alzheimer type, senile onset, with delusions
290.21	Primary degenerative dementia of the Alzheimer type, senile onset, with depression

290.30	Primary degenerative dementia of the Alzheimer type, senile onset, with delirium
290.40	Multi-infarct dementia, uncomplicated
290.41	Multi-infarct dementia, with delirium
290.42	Multi-infarct dementia, with delusions
290.43	Multi-infarct dementia, with depression
291.00	Alcohol withdrawal delirium
291.10	Alcohol amnestic disorder
291.20	Dementia associated with alcoholism
291.30	Alcohol hallucinosis
291.40	Alcohol idiosyncratic intoxication
291.80	Uncomplicated alcohol withdrawal
292.00	Amphetamine or similarly acting sympathomimetic withdrawal
292.00	Cocaine withdrawal
292.00	Nicotine withdrawal
292.00	Opioid withdrawal
292.00	Other or unspecified psychoactive substance withdrawal
292.00	Sedative, hypnotic, or anxiolytic withdrawal delirium
292.00	Uncomplicated sedative, hypnotic, or anxiolytic withdrawal
292.11	Amphetamine or similarly acting sympathomimetic delusional disorder
292.11	Cannabis delusional disorder
292.11	Cocaine delusional disorder
292.11	Hallucinogen delusional disorder
292.11	Other or unspecified psychoactive substance delusional disorder
292.11	Phencyclidine (PCP) or similarly acting arylcyclohexylamine delusional disorder
292.12	Other or unspecified psychoactive substance hallucinosis
292.81	Amphetamine or similarly acting sympathomimetic delirium

292.81	Cocaine delirium
292.81	Other or unspecified psychoactive substance delirium
292.81	Phencyclidine (PCP) or similarly acting arylcyclohexylamine delirium
292.82	Other or unspecified psychoactive substance dementia
292.83	Other or unspecified psychoactive substance amnestic disorder
292.83	Sedative, hypnotic, or anxiolytic amnestic disorder
292.84	Hallucinogen mood disorder
292.84	Other or unspecified psychoactive substance mood disorder
292.84	Phencyclidine (PCP) or similarly acting arylcyclohexylamine mood disorder
292.89	Other or unspecified psychoactive substance anxiety disorder
292.89	Other or unspecified psychoactive substance personality disorder
292.89	Posthallucinogen perception disorder
292.90	Other or unspecified psychoactive substance organic mental disorder NOS
292.90	Phencyclidine (PCP) or similarly acting arylcyclohexylamine organic mental disorder NOS
293.00	Delirium (etiology noted on Axis III or is unknown)
293.81	Organic delusional disorder (etiology noted on Axis III or is unknown)
293.82	Organic hallucinosis (etiology noted on Axis III or is unknown)
293.83	Organic mood disorder (etiology noted on Axis III or is unknown)
294.00	Amnestic disorder (etiology noted on Axis III or is unknown)
294.10	Dementia (etiology noted on Axis III or is unknown)

294.80	Organic anxiety disorder (etiology noted on Axis III or is unknown)
294.80	Organic mental disorder NOS (etiology noted on Axis III or is unknown)
295.10	Schizophrenia, disorganized type, unspecified
295.11	Schizophrenia, disorganized type, subchronic
295.12	Schizophrenia, disorganized type, chronic
295.13	Schizophrenia, disorganized type, subchronic with acute exacerbation
295.14	Schizophrenia, disorganized type, chronic with acute exacerbation
295.20	Schizophrenia, catatonic type, unspecified
295.21	Schizophrenia, catatonic type, subchronic
295.22	Schizophrenia, catatonic type, chronic
295.23	Schizophrenia, catatonic type, subchronic with acute exacerbation
295.24	Schizophrenia, catatonic type, chronic with acute exacerbation
295.30	Schizophrenia, paranoid type, unspecified
295.31	Schizophrenia, paranoid type, subchronic
295.32	Schizophrenia, paranoid type, chronic
295.33	Schizophrenia, paranoid type, subchronic with acute exacerbation
295.34	Schizophrenia, paranoid type, chronic with acute exacerbation
295.40	Schizophreniform disorder
295.60	Schizophrenia, residual type, unspecified
295.61	Schizophrenia, residual type, subchronic
295.62	Schizophrenia, residual type, chronic
295.63	Schizophrenia, residual type, subchronic with acute exacerbation
295.64	Schizophrenia, residual type, chronic with acute exacerbation
295.70	Schizoaffective disorder

295.91	Schizophrenia, undifferentiated type, subchronic
295.92	Schizophrenia, undifferentiated type, chronic
295.93	Schizophrenia, undifferentiated type, subchronic with acute exacerbation
295.94	Schizophrenia, undifferentiated type, chronic with acute exacerbation
295.95	Schizophrenia, undifferentiated type, unspecified
296.20	Major depression, single episode, unspecified
296.21	Major depression, single episode, mild
296.22	Major depression, single episode, moderate
296.23	Major depression, single episode, severe, without psychotic features
296.24	Major depression, single episode, with psychotic features
296.25	Major depression, single episode, in partial remission
296.26	Major depression, single episode, in full remission
296.30	Major depression, recurrent, unspecified
296.31	Major depression, recurrent, mild
296.32	Major depression, recurrent, moderate
296.33	Major depression, recurrent, severe, without psychotic features
296.34	Major depression, recurrent, with psychotic features
296.35	Major depression, recurrent, in partial remission
296.36	Major depression, recurrent, in full remission
296.40	Bipolar disorder, manic, unspecified
296.41	Bipolar disorder, manic, mild
296.42	Bipolar disorder, manic, moderate

296.43	Bipolar disorder, manic, severe, without psychotic features
296.44	Bipolar disorder, manic, with psychotic features
296.45	Bipolar disorder, manic, in partial remission
296.46	Bipolar disorder, manic, in full remission
296.50	Bipolar disorder, depressed, unspecified
296.51	Bipolar disorder, depressed, mild
296.52	Bipolar disorder, depressed, moderate
296.53	Bipolar disorder, depressed, severe, without psychotic features
296.54	Bipolar disorder, depressed, with psychotic features
296.55	Bipolar disorder, depressed, in partial remission
296.56	Bipolar disorder, depressed, in full remission
296.60	Bipolar disorder, mixed, unspecified
296.61	Bipolar disorder, mixed, mild
296.62	Bipolar disorder, mixed, moderate
296.63	Bipolar disorder, mixed, severe, without psychotic features
296.64	Bipolar disorder, mixed, with psychotic features
296.65	Bipolar disorder, mixed, in partial remission
296.66	Bipolar disorder, mixed, in full remission
296.70	Bipolar disorder NOS
297.10	Delusional disorder
297.30	Induced psychotic disorder
298.80	Brief reactive psychosis
298.90	Psychotic disorder NOS
299.00	Autistic disorder
299.80	Pervasive developmental disorder NOS
300.00	Anxiety disorder NOS
300.01	Panic disorder, without agoraphobia

300.02	Generalized anxiety disorder
300.11	Conversion disorder
300.12	Psychogenic amnesia
300.13	Psychogenic fugue
300.14	Multiple personality disorder
300.15	Dissociative disorder NOS
300.16	Factitious disorder with psychological symptoms
300.19	Factitious disorder NOS
300.21	Panic disorder, with agoraphobia
300.22	Agoraphobia without history of panic disorder
300.23	Social phobia
300.29	Simple phobia
300.30	Obsessive compulsive disorder
300.40	Dysthymia
300.60	Depersonalization disorder
300.70	Body dysmorphic disorder
300.70	Hypochondriasis
300.70	Somatoform disorder NOS
300.70	Undifferentiated somatoform disorder
300.81	Somatization disorder
300.90	Unspecified mental disorder (nonpsychotic)
301.00	Paranoid personality disorder
301.13	Cyclothymia
301.20	Schizoid personality disorder
301.22	Schizotypal personality disorder
301.40	Obsessive compulsive personality disorder
301.50	Histrionic personality disorder
301.51	Factitious disorder with physical symptoms
301.60	Dependent personality disorder
301.70	Antisocial personality disorder
301.81	Narcissistic personality disorder
301.82	Avoidant personality disorder
301.83	Borderline personality disorder

301.84	Passive aggressive personality disorder
301.90	Personality disorder NOS
302.20	Pedophilia
302.30	Transvestic fetishism
302.40	Exhibitionism
302.50	Transsexualism
302.60	Gender identity disorder of childhood
302.70	Sexual dysfunction NOS
302.71	Hypoactive sexual desire disorder
⎡ 302.72	Female sexual arousal disorder
⎣ 302.72	Male erectile disorder
302.73	Inhibited female orgasm
302.74	Inhibited male orgasm
302.75	Premature ejaculation
302.76	Dyspareunia
302.79	Sexual aversion disorder
302.81	Fetishism
302.82	Voyeurism
302.83	Sexual masochism
302.84	Sexual sadism
⎡ 302.85	Gender identity disorder NOS
⎣ 302.85	Gender identity disorder of adolescence or adulthood, nontranssexual type
302.89	Frotteurism
⎡ 302.90	Sexual disorder NOS
⎣ 302.90	Paraphilia NOS
303.00	Alcohol intoxication
303.90	Alcohol dependence
304.00	Opioid dependence
304.10	Sedative, hypnotic, or anxiolytic dependence
304.20	Cocaine dependence
304.30	Cannabis dependence
304.40	Amphetamine or similarly acting sympathomimetic dependence
⎡ 304.50	Hallucinogen dependence
⎣ 304.50	Phencyclidine (PCP) or similarly acting arylcyclohexylamine dependence

304.60	Inhalant dependence
⌈ 304.90	Polysubstance dependence
⌊ 304.90	Psychoactive substance dependence NOS
305.00	Alcohol abuse
305.10	Nicotine dependence
⌈ 305.20	Cannabis abuse
⌊ 305.20	Cannabis intoxication
⌈ 305.30	Hallucinogen abuse
⌊ 305.30	Hallucinogen hallucinosis
⌈ 305.40	Sedative, hypnotic, or anxiolytic abuse
305.40	Sedative, hypnotic, or anxiolytic intoxication
⌈ 305.50	Opioid abuse
⌊ 305.50	Opioid intoxication
⌈ 305.60	Cocaine abuse
⌊ 305.60	Cocaine intoxication
⌈ 305.70	Amphetamine or similarly acting sympathomimetic abuse
305.70	Amphetamine or similarly acting sympathomimetic intoxication
⌈ 305.90	Caffeine intoxication
305.90	Inhalant abuse
305.90	Inhalant intoxication
305.90	Other or unspecified psychoactive substance intoxication
305.90	Phencyclidine (PCP) or similarly acting arylcyclohexylamine abuse
305.90	Phencyclidine (PCP) or similarly acting arylcyclohexylamine intoxication
305.90	Polysubstance abuse
⌊ 305.90	Psychoactive substance abuse NOS
306.51	Vaginismus
⌈ 307.00	Cluttering
⌊ 307.00	Stuttering
307.10	Anorexia nervosa
307.20	Tic disorder NOS
307.21	Transient tic disorder
307.22	Chronic motor or vocal tic disorder

307.23	Tourette's disorder
307.30	Stereotypy/habit disorder
⎡ 307.40	Dyssomnia NOS
⎣ 307.40	Parasomnia NOS
⎡ 307.42	Insomnia related to another mental disorder (nonorganic)
⎣ 307.42	Primary insomnia
307.44	Hypersomnia related to another mental disorder (nonorganic)
307.45	Sleep-wake schedule disorder
⎡ 307.46	Sleep terror disorder
⎣ 307.46	Sleepwalking disorder
307.47	Dream anxiety disorder (Nightmare disorder)
307.50	Eating Disorder NOS
307.51	Bulimia nervosa
307.52	Pica
307.53	Rumination disorder of infancy
307.60	Functional enuresis
307.70	Functional encopresis
307.80	Somatoform pain disorder
307.90	Late luteal phase dysphoric disorder
309.00	Adjustment disorder with depressed mood
309.21	Separation anxiety disorder
309.23	Adjustment disorder with work (or academic) inhibition
309.24	Adjustment disorder with anxious mood
309.28	Adjustment disorder with mixed emotional features
309.30	Adjustment disorder with disturbance of conduct
309.40	Adjustment disorder with mixed disturbance of emotions and conduct
309.82	Adjustment disorder with physical complaints
309.83	Adjustment disorder with withdrawal
309.89	Post-traumatic stress disorder

309.90	Adjustment disorder NOS
310.10	Organic personality disorder (etiology noted on Axis III or is unknown)
311.00	Depressive disorder NOS
312.00	Conduct disorder, solitary aggressive type
312.20	Conduct disorder, group type
312.31	Pathological gambling
312.32	Kleptomania
312.33	Pyromania
312.34	Intermittent explosive disorder
⌈ 312.39	Impulse control disorder NOS
⌊ 312.39	Trichotillomania
312.90	Conduct disorder, undifferentiated type
313.00	Overanxious disorder
313.21	Avoidant disorder of childhood or adolescence
313.23	Elective mutism
313.81	Oppositional defiant disorder
313.82	Identity disorder
313.89	Reactive attachment disorder of infancy or early childhood
314.00	Undifferentiated attention-deficit disorder
314.01	Attention-deficit hyperactivity disorder
315.00	Developmental reading disorder
315.10	Developmental arithmetic disorder
⌈ 315.31	Developmental expressive language disorder
⌊ 315.31	Developmental receptive language disorder
315.39	Developmental articulation disorder
315.40	Developmental coordination disorder
315.80	Developmental expressive writing disorder
⌈ 315.90	Developmental disorder NOS
⌊ 315.90	Specific developmental disorder NOS
316.00	Psychological factors affecting physical condition
317.00	Mild mental retardation
318.00	Moderate mental retardation

318.10	Severe mental retardation
318.20	Profound mental retardation
319.00	Unspecified mental retardation
⎡ 780.50	Hypersomnia related to a known organic factor
⎣ 780.50	Insomnia related to a known organic factor
780.54	Primary hypersomnia
⎡ 799.90	Diagnosis or condition deferred on Axis I
⎣ 799.90	Diagnosis or condition deferred on Axis II
V15.81	Noncompliance with medical treatment
V40.00	Borderline intellectual functioning
V61.10	Marital problem
V61.20	Parent-child problem
V61.80	Other specified family circumstances
V62.20	Occupational problem
V62.30	Academic problem
V62.81	Other interpersonal problem
V62.82	Uncomplicated bereavement
V62.89	Phase of life problem or other life circumstance problem
V65.20	Malingering
V71.01	Adult antisocial behavior
V71.02	Childhood or adolescent antisocial behavior
⎡ V71.09	No diagnosis or condition on Axis I
⎣ V71.09	No diagnosis or condition on Axis II

Abbreviated Symptom Index: Index of Selected Symptoms Included in the Diagnostic Criteria

Abbreviated Symptom Index:
Index of Selected Symptoms
Included in the Diagnostic Criteria
(Abridged from index in DSM-III-R)[1]

The purpose of this index is to identify those diagnostic criteria in the various disorders that refer, either precisely or in a more general way, to a particular symptom. For example, this index lists 21 disorders that have a criterion that refers in some way to *decreased energy*. In the index, the name of each disorder is followed by the letter or number of the criterion that refers to the symptom. For example, among the disorders listed under *decreased energy* is "Dysthymia: B(3)," which indicates that criterion B(3) in the diagnostic criteria for Dysthymia refers to decreased energy.

Since the significance of any given clinical finding has to be weighed within the total context of the person's history and presentation, this index should not be the basis for making a differential diagnosis. In the above example, although 21 disorders include the symptom *decreased energy*, the importance of this symptom is quite variable from one disorder to another.

Often a disorder is listed whose criteria do not directly mention the indexing symptom. For example, Schizoaffective Disorder is listed under *psychomotor retardation*, although this symptom is not directly

---

[1] Prepared by Michael B. First, M.D., and Robert L. Spitzer, M.D.

However, *psychomotor retardation* is referred to in criterion A(5) for Major Depressive Episode, which is mentioned in Criterion A for Schizoaffective Disorder, and is therefore *indirectly* referred to in the criteria for Schizoaffective Disorder. When the criterion for a disorder refers to a symptom only indirectly, the direct reference to the symptom is included in brackets. In the above example, the index entry "Schizoaffective disorder: A [see Major depressive episode: A(5)]" indicates that *psychomotor retardation* is indirectly referred to in criterion A of Schizoaffective Disorder, but is directly referred to in criterion A(5) of Major Depressive Episode.

It should be noted that this index deals only with symptoms that appear in the DSM-III-R diagnostic criteria; it does not index associated features. The list for a particular symptom is therefore limited to diagnoses in which the symptom is (directly or indirectly) part of the defining criteria for the disorder. For example, although *depressed mood* is often associated with Schizophrenia, Schizophrenia is not listed under *depressed mood* because this symptom does not appear in the diagnostic criteria for Schizophrenia. In addition, the residual disorders within each major diagnostic class (for example, Eating Disorder Not Otherwise Specified) are not listed in the index.

Use of the Index. The symptoms are organized into the following symptom groups:

I.   ACTIVITY
II.   ANXIETY SYMPTOMS
III.   BEHAVIOR
IV.   COGNITION/MEMORY/ATTENTION
V.   EATING DISTURBANCE
VI.   ENERGY
VII.   FORM AND AMOUNT OF THOUGHT/SPEECH

VIII.   MOOD/AFFECT DISTURBANCE
IX.   PERCEPTUAL DISTURBANCE
X.   PHYSICAL SIGNS AND SYMPTOMS
XI.   SLEEP DISTURBANCE
XII.   THOUGHT CONTENT (INCLUDING
       DELUSIONS)

The clinician should first consult these symptom groups to select the one most likely to include the symptom under consideration. Usually, the choice of symptom group will be clear. Symptoms that cannot be clearly categorized by a single group are listed in several groups. For example, *grandiosity* is listed under MOOD/AFFECT DISTURBANCE, THOUGHT CONTENT, and PERSONALITY TRAITS. Listed after each symptom is a page number that indicates where in this appendix the list of indexed diagnoses can be found.

An example of how to use this appendix follows:

1. The clinician is interested in determining all of the disorders that have as one of their defining features the symptom "repeated awakening in the middle of the night."

2. The clinician consults the list of symptom groups above and decides that "repeated awakening in the middle of the night" will most likely be listed under SLEEP DISTURBANCE.

3. The clinician looks up SLEEP DISTURBANCE and finds that the most likely listed sleep symptom that corresponds to "repeated awakening in the middle of the night" is *insomnia*. The clinician then turns to the page number following the word *insomnia* and finds the list of disorders whose diagnostic criteria refer to *insomnia*.

4. The clinician then turns to the Index of Diagnostic Terms to locate the page number on which the diagnosis is described or on which the criteria for that diagnosis appears.

List of Selected Symptoms

I. ACTIVITY
    catatonia p. 270
    psychomotor agitation p. 271
    psychomotor retardation p. 272

II. ANXIETY SYMPTOMS
    avoidance behavior p. 276
    fear of embarrassment due to a physical
        symptom p. 273
    fear of social situations p. 274
    worrying p. 274

III. BEHAVIOR
    aggression or rage p. 274
    antisocial behavior p. 275
    apathy p. 283
    avoidance behavior p. 276
    catatonia p. 270
    suicide attempt p. 276

IV. COGNITION/MEMORY/ATTENTION
    distractibility p. 277
    impaired judgment p. 278
    memory impairment p. 279

V. EATING DISTURBANCE
    decreased appetite p. 279
    increased appetite p. 280

VI. ENERGY
decrease in energy or fatigue p. 281

VII. FORM AND AMOUNT OF THOUGHT/SPEECH
abnormalities in the production of speech
p. 282
flight of ideas p. 282
incoherence or loosening of associations
p. 282
pressured speech p. 283

VIII. MOOD/AFFECT DISTURBANCE
apathy p. 283
blunted affect p. 284
depressed mood p. 284
elevated mood p. 285
flat affect p. 286
grandiosity p. 302
hopelessness p. 302
irritable mood or irritability (in adults) p. 286
irritable mood or irritability (in children and
adolescents) p. 287
marked mood shifts p. 289

IX. PERCEPTUAL DISTURBANCE
hallucinations p. 289
illusions or perceptual distortions p. 290

X. PHYSICAL SIGNS AND SYMPTOMS
autonomic
elevated blood pressure p. 291
pupillary constriction p. 291
pupillary dilation p. 291
sweating p. 291
tachycardia p. 292
cardiovascular
chest pain p. 293

elevated blood pressure p. 291
tachycardia p. 292
gastrointestinal
abdominal pain p. 293
diarrhea p. 294
vomiting p. 294
neurologic
gait abnormalities p. 295
nystagmus p. 295
paralysis p. 295
tremor or trembling p. 296
physical complaint without organic pathology
p. 296

XI. SLEEP DISTURBANCE
hypersomnia p. 296
insomnia p. 298

XII. THOUGHT CONTENT (INCLUDING
DELUSIONS)
delusions
bizarre delusions p. 299
nonbizarre delusions p. 300
grandiosity p. 302
hopelessness p. 302
ideas of reference p. 303
paranoid ideation (nondelusional) p. 303
suicidal ideation p. 304

Index of Diagnostic Criteria

catatonia
　　　Bipolar disorder, depressed: B [see Major depressive episode with psychotic features]
　　　Bipolar disorder, manic: A [see Manic episode with mood-incongruent psychotic features: (b)]
　　　Bipolar disorder, mixed: A [see Major depressive episode with psychotic features or Manic episode with mood-incongruent psychotic features: (b)]
　　　Brief reactive psychosis: A(4)
　　　Hallucinogen mood disorder: A [see Major depressive episode with psychotic features or Manic episode with mood-incongruent psychotic features: (b)]
　　　Major depression, single or recurrent episode: A [see Major depressive episode with psychotic features]
　　　Multi-infarct dementia with depression [see Major depressive episode with psychotic features]
　　　Organic mood syndrome: A [see Major depressive episode with psychotic features or Manic episode with mood-incongruent psychotic features: (b)]
　　　Phencyclidine (PCP) or similarly acting arylcyclohexylamine mood disorder: A [see Major de-

pressive episode with psychotic features or Manic episode with mood-incongruent psychotic features: (b)]

Primary degenerative dementia of the Alzheimer type with depression [see Major depressive episode with psychotic features]

Schizoaffective disorder: A [see Major depressive episode with psychotic features or Manic episode with mood-incongruent psychotic features: (b) or Schizophrenia: A(1)(d)]

Schizophrenia: A(1)(d)

Schizophreniform disorder: A [see Schizophrenia: A(1)(d)]

psychomotor agitation

Alcohol withdrawal delirium: A [see Delirium: C(4)]

Amphetamine or similarly acting sympathomimetic delirium: A [see Delirium: C(4)]

Amphetamine or similarly acting sympathomimetic intoxication: B

Amphetamine or similarly acting sympathomimetic withdrawal: A(3)

Bipolar disorder, depressed: B [see Major depressive episode: A(5)]

Bipolar disorder, manic: A [see Manic episode: B(6)]

Bipolar disorder, mixed: A [see Major depressive episode: A(5) or Manic episode: B(6)]

Caffeine intoxication: B(12)

Cocaine delirium: A [see Delirium: C(4)]

Cocaine intoxication: B

Cocaine withdrawal: A(3)

Cyclothymia: A [see Hypomanic/Manic episode: B(6)]

Delirium: C(4)

Hallucinogen mood disorder: A [see Major depressive episode: A(5) or Manic episode: B(6)]

Inhalant intoxication: B

Major depression, single or recurrent episode: A [see Major depressive episode: A(5)]

Major depressive episode, melancholic type: (5)

Multi-infarct dementia with delirium [see Delirium: C(4)]

Multi-infarct dementia with depression [see Major depressive episode: A(5)]

Organic mood syndrome: A [see Major depressive episode: A(5) or Manic episode: B(6)]

Phencyclidine (PCP) or similarly acting arylcyclohexylamine delirium: A [see Delirium: C(4)]

Phencyclidine (PCP) or similarly acting arylcyclohexylamine intoxication: B

Phencyclidine (PCP) or similarly acting arylcyclohexylamine mood disorder: A [see Major depressive episode: A(5) or Manic episode: B(6)]

Primary degenerative dementia of the Alzheimer type with delirium [see Delirium: C(4)]

Primary degenerative dementia of the Alzheimer type with depression [see Major depressive episode: A(5)]

Schizoaffective disorder: A [see Major depressive episode: A(5) or Manic episode: B(6)]

Sedative, hypnotic, or anxiolytic withdrawal delirium: A [see Delirium: C(4)]

psychomotor retardation

Alcohol withdrawal delirium: A [see Delirium: C(4)]

Amphetamine or similarly acting sympathomimetic delirium: A [see Delirium: C(4)]

Bipolar disorder, depressed: B [see Major depressive episode: A(5)]

Bipolar disorder, mixed: A [see Major depressive episode: A(5)]

Cocaine delirium: A [see Delirium: C(4)]

Delirium: C(4)

Hallucinogen mood disorder: A [see Major depressive episode: A(5)]

Inhalant intoxication: C(8)

Major depression, single or recurrent episode: A [see Major depressive episode: A(5)]

Major depressive episode, melancholic type: (5)

Multi-infarct dementia with delirium [see Delirium: C(4)]

Multi-infarct dementia with depression [see Major depressive episode: A(5)]

Opioid intoxication: B

Organic mood syndrome: A [see Major depressive episode: A(5)]

Phencyclidine (PCP) or similarly acting arylcyclohexylamine delirium: A [see Delirium: C(4)]

Phencyclidine (PCP) or similarly acting arylcyclohexylamine mood disorder: A [see Major depressive episode: A(5)]

Primary degenerative dementia of the Alzheimer type with delirium [see Delirium: C(4)]

Primary degenerative dementia of the Alzheimer type with depression [see Major depressive episode: A(5)]

Schizoaffective disorder: A [see Major depressive episode: A(5)]

Sedative, hypnotic, or anxiolytic withdrawal delirium: A [see Delirium: C(4)]

fear of embarrassment due to physical symptoms
Agoraphobia without history of panic disorder: A

Body dysmorphic disorder: A
Panic disorder with agoraphobia: B
Social phobia: A

fear of social situations
    Avoidant disorder of childhood or adolescence:
        A
    Avoidant personality disorder: (5)
    Schizotypal personality disorder: A(2)
    Social phobia: A

excessive worrying
    Adjustment disorder with anxious mood
    Adjustment disorder with mixed disturbance of
        emotions and conduct
    Adjustment disorder with mixed emotional fea-
        tures
    Generalized anxiety disorder: A
    Organic anxiety syndrome: A [see Generalized
        anxiety disorder: A]
    Overanxious disorder: A
    Separation anxiety disorder: A(1)

outbursts of aggression or rage
    Alcohol idiosyncratic intoxication: A
    Alcohol intoxication: B
    Amphetamine or similarly acting sympatho-
        mimetic intoxication: B
    Antisocial personality disorder: C(3)
    Borderline personality disorder: (4)
    Cocaine intoxication: B
    Dementia: B(4)
    Dementia associated with alcoholism: A [see De-
        mentia: B(4)]
    Inhalant intoxication: B
    Intermittent explosive disorder: A
    Late luteal phase dysphoric disorder: B(2)

Mental retardation: B
Multi-infarct dementia: A [see Dementia: B(4)]
Nicotine withdrawal: B(2)
Oppositional defiant disorder: A(7)
Organic personality syndrome: A(2)
Post-traumatic stress disorder: D(2)
Primary degenerative dementia of the Alzheimer
    type: A [see Dementia: B(4)]
Sedative, hypnotic, or anxiolytic intoxication: B

antisocial behavior
    Adjustment disorder with disturbance of conduct
    Adjustment disorder with mixed disturbance of
        emotions and conduct
    Adult antisocial behavior
    Antisocial personality disorder: C(2)
    Bipolar disorder, manic: A [see Manic episode:
        B(7)]
    Bipolar disorder, mixed: A [see Manic episode:
        B(7)]
    Borderline personality disorder: (2)
    Childhood or adolescent antisocial behavior
    Conduct disorder: A
    Cyclothymia: A [see Hypomanic/Manic episode:
        B(7)]
    Hallucinogen mood disorder: A [see Manic epi-
        sode: B(7)]
    Intermittent explosive disorder: A
    Kleptomania: A
    Organic mood syndrome: A [see Manic episode:
        B(7)]
    Phencyclidine (PCP) or similarly acting arylcyclo-
        hexylamine mood disorder: A [see Manic
        episode: B(7)]
    Pyromania: A
    Schizoaffective disorder: A [see Manic episode:
        B(7)]

avoidance behavior

> Agoraphobia without history of panic disorder: A
> Avoidant disorder of childhood or adolescence:
> A
> Avoidant personality disorder: (4)
> Borderline personality disorder: (8)
> Dependent personality disorder: (6)
> Panic disorder with agoraphobia: B
> Post-traumatic stress disorder: C(2)
> Separation anxiety disorder: A(5)
> Sexual aversion disorder: A
> Simple phobia: C
> Social phobia: D

suicide attempt

> Bipolar disorder, depressed: B [see Major depressive episode: A(9)]
> Bipolar disorder, mixed: A [see Major depressive episode: A(9)]
> Borderline personality disorder: (5)
> Hallucinogen mood disorder: A [see Major depressive episode: A(9)]
> Major depression, single or recurrent episode: A [see Major depressive episode: A(9)]
> Multi-infarct dementia with depression [see Major depressive episode: A(9)]
> Organic mood syndrome: A [see Major depressive episode: A(9)]
> Phencyclidine (PCP) or similarly acting arylcyclohexylamine mood disorder: A [see Major depressive episode: A(9)]
> Primary degenerative dementia of the Alzheimer type with depression [see Major depressive episode: A(9)]
> Schizoaffective disorder: A [see Major depressive episode: A(9)]

distractibility

> Alcohol withdrawal delirium: A [see Delirium: A]
>
> Amphetamine or similarly acting sympatho-mimetic
>
> delirium: A [see Delirium: A]
>
> Attention-deficit hyperactivity disorder: A(3)
>
> Bipolar disorder, manic: A [see Manic episode: B(5)]
>
> Bipolar disorder, mixed: A [see Manic episode: B(5)]
>
> Cocaine delirium: A [see Delirium: A]
>
> Cyclothymia: A [see Hypomanic/Manic episode: B(5)]
>
> Delirium: A
>
> Hallucinogen mood disorder: A [see Manic episode: B(5)]
>
> Multi-infarct dementia with delirium [see Delirium: A]
>
> Opioid intoxication: C(3)
>
> Organic mood syndrome: A [see Manic episode: B(5)]
>
> Phencyclidine (PCP) or similarly acting arylcyclo-hexylamine delirium: A [see Delirium: A]
>
> Phencyclidine (PCP) or similarly acting arylcyclo-hexylamine mood disorder: A [see Manic episode: B(5)]
>
> Primary degenerative dementia of the Alzheimer type with delirium [see Delirium: A]
>
> Schizoaffective disorder: A [see Manic episode: B(5)]
>
> Sedative, hypnotic, or anxiolytic intoxication: C(4)
>
> Sedative, hypnotic, or anxiolytic withdrawal delir-ium: A [see Delirium: A]
>
> Undifferentiated attention-deficit disorder

impaired judgment
    Alcohol intoxication: B
    Amphetamine or similarly acting sympatho-
        mimetic intoxication: B
    Attention-deficit hyperactivity disorder: A(14)
    Bipolar disorder, manic: A [see Manic episode:
        B(7)]
    Bipolar disorder, mixed: A [see Manic episode:
        B(7)]
    Borderline personality disorder: (2)
    Cannabis intoxication: B
    Cocaine intoxication: B
    Cyclothymia: A [see Hypomanic/Manic episode:
        B(7)]
    Dementia: B(2)
    Dementia associated with alcoholism: A [see De-
        mentia: B(2)]
    Hallucinogen hallucinosis: B
    Hallucinogen mood disorder: A [see Manic epi-
        sode: B(7)]
    Inhalant intoxication: B
    Mental retardation: B
    Multi-infarct dementia: A [see Dementia: B(2)]
    Opioid intoxication: B
    Organic mood syndrome: A [see Manic episode:
        B(7)]
    Organic personality syndrome: A(3)
    Phencyclidine (PCP) or similarly acting arylcyclo-
        hexylamine intoxication: B
    Phencyclidine (PCP) or similarly acting arylcyclo-
        hexylamine mood disorder: A [see Manic
        episode: B(7)]
    Primary degenerative dementia of the Alzheimer
        type: A [see Dementia: B(2)]
    Schizoaffective disorder: A [see Manic episode:
        B(7)]
    Sedative, hypnotic, or anxiolytic intoxication: B

memory impairment

    Alcohol amnestic disorder: A [see Amnestic syndrome: A]

    Alcohol withdrawal delirium: A [see Delirium: C(6)]

    Amnestic syndrome: A

    Amphetamine or similarly acting sympathomimetic delirium: A [see Delirium: C(6)]

    Cocaine delirium: A [see Delirium: C(6)]

    Conversion disorder: A

    Delirium: C(6)

    Dementia: A

    Dementia associated with alcoholism: A [see Dementia: A]

    Multi-infarct dementia with delirium [see Delirium: C(6) or Dementia: A]

    Opioid intoxication: C(3)

    Phencyclidine (PCP) or similarly acting arylcyclohexylamine delirium: A [see Delirium: C(6)]

    Primary degenerative dementia of the Alzheimer type, with delirium [see Delirium: C(6) or Dementia: A]

    Sedative, hypnotic, or anxiolytic amnestic disorder: A [see Amnestic syndrome: A]

    Sedative, hypnotic, or anxiolytic intoxication: C(4)

    Sedative, hypnotic, or anxiolytic withdrawal delirium: A [see Delirium: C(6)]

decreased appetite

    Adjustment disorder with depressed mood

    Bipolar disorder, depressed: B [see Major depressive episode: A(3)]

    Bipolar disorder, mixed: A [see Major depressive episode: A(3)]

    Dysthymia: B(1)

Hallucinogen mood disorder: A [see Major depressive episode: A(3)]

Major depression, single or recurrent episode: A [see Major depressive episode: A(3)]

Multi-infarct dementia with depression [see Major depressive episode: A(3)]

Organic mood syndrome: A [see Major depressive episode: A(3)]

Phencyclidine (PCP) or similarly acting arylcyclohexylamine mood disorder: A [see Major depressive episode: A(3)]

Primary degenerative dementia of the Alzheimer type with depression [see Major depressive episode: A(3)]

Schizoaffective disorder: A [see Major depressive episode: A(3)]

Uncomplicated bereavement

increased appetite

Adjustment disorder with depressed mood

Bipolar disorder, depressed: B [see Major depressive episode: A(3)]

Bipolar disorder, mixed: A [see Major depressive episode: A(3)]

Cannabis intoxication: C(2)

Dysthymia: B(1)

Hallucinogen mood disorder: A [see Major depressive episode: A(3)]

Late luteal phase dysphoric disorder: B(8)

Major depression, single or recurrent episode: A [see Major depressive episode: A(3)]

Multi-infarct dementia with depression [see Major depressive episode: A(3)]

Nicotine withdrawal: B(7)

Organic mood syndrome: A [see Major depressive episode: A(3)]

Phencyclidine (PCP) or similarly acting arylcyclo-hexylamine mood disorder: A [see Major depressive episode: A(3)]

Primary degenerative dementia of the Alzheimer type with depression [see Major depressive episode: A(3)]

Schizoaffective disorder: A [see Major depressive episode: A(3)]

Uncomplicated bereavement

decrease in energy or fatigue

Adjustment disorder with depressed mood

Amphetamine or similarly acting sympatho-mimetic withdrawal: A(1)

Bipolar disorder, depressed: B [see Major depressive episode: A(6)]

Bipolar disorder, mixed: A [see Major depressive episode: A(6)]

Cocaine withdrawal: A(1)

Dysthymia: B(3)

Hallucinogen mood disorder: A [see Major depressive episode: A(6)]

Inhalant intoxication: C(6)

Insomnia disorder: B

Late luteal phase dysphoric disorder: B(6)

Major depression, single or recurrent episode: A [see Major depressive episode: A(6)]

Multi-infarct dementia with depression [see Major depressive episode: A(6)]

Organic mood syndrome: A [see Major depressive episode: A(6)]

Phencyclidine (PCP) or similarly acting arylcyclo-hexylamine mood disorder: A [see Major depressive episode: A(6)]

Primary degenerative dementia of the Alzheimer type with depression [see Major depressive episode: A(6)]

Schizoaffective disorder: A [see Major depressive episode: A(6)]

Schizophrenia: D(9)

Sleep-Wake schedule disorder: A [see Insomnia disorder: B]

Uncomplicated alcohol withdrawal: A(2)

Uncomplicated bereavement

Uncomplicated sedative, hypnotic, or anxiolytic withdrawal: A(2)

marked abnormalities in the production of speech

Autistic disorder: B(4)

Cluttering

Stuttering

flight of ideas

Bipolar disorder, manic: A [see Manic episode: B(4)]

Bipolar disorder, mixed: A [see Manic episode: B(4)]

Cyclothymia: A [see Hypomanic/Manic episode: B(4)]

Hallucinogen mood disorder: A [see Manic episode: B(4)]

Organic mood syndrome: A [see Manic episode: B(4)]

Phencyclidine (PCP) or similarly acting arylcyclohexylamine mood disorder: A [see Manic episode: B(4)]

Schizoaffective disorder: A [see Manic episode: B(4)]

incoherence or loosening of associations

Alcohol withdrawal delirium: A [see Delirium: B]

Amphetamine or similarly acting sympathomimetic delirium: A [see Delirium: B]

Brief reactive psychosis: A(1)

Cocaine delirium: A [see Delirium: B]

Delirium: B

Multi-infarct dementia with delirium [see Delirium: B]

Phencyclidine (PCP) or similarly acting arylcyclohexylamine delirium: A [see Delirium: B]

Primary degenerative dementia of the Alzheimer type with delirium [see Delirium: B]

Schizoaffective disorder: A [see Schizophrenia: A(1)(c)]

Schizophrenia: A(1)(c)

Schizophrenia, disorganized type: A

Schizophrenia, undifferentiated type: A

Schizophreniform disorder: A [see Schizophrenia: A(1)(c)]

Sedative, hypnotic, or anxiolytic withdrawal delirium: A [see Delirium: B]

pressured speech

Bipolar disorder, manic: A [see Manic episode: B(3)]

Bipolar disorder, mixed: A [see Manic episode: B(3)]

Cyclothymia: A [see Hypomanic/Manic episode: B(3)]

Hallucinogen mood disorder: A [see Manic episode: B(3)]

Organic mood syndrome: A [see Manic episode: B(3)]

Phencyclidine (PCP) or similarly acting arylcyclohexylamine mood disorder: A [see Manic episode: B(3)]

Schizoaffective disorder: A [see Manic episode: B(3)]

apathy

Bipolar disorder, depressed: B [see Major depressive episode: A(2)]

Bipolar disorder, mixed: A [see Major depressive episode: A(2)]

Dementia: B(4)

Dementia associated with alcoholism [see Dementia: B(4)]

Hallucinogen mood disorder: A [see Major depressive episode: A(2)]

Inhalant intoxication: B

Major depression, single or recurrent episode: A [see Major depressive episode: A(2)]

Major depressive episode, melancholic type: (1)

Multi-infarct dementia with depression [see Dementia: B(4) or Major depressive episode: A(2)]

Opioid intoxication: B

Organic mood syndrome: A [see Major depressive episode: A(2)]

Organic personality syndrome: A(4)

Phencyclidine (PCP) or similarly acting arylcyclohexylamine mood disorder: A [see Major depressive episode: A(2)]

Post-traumatic stress disorder: C(4)

Primary degenerative dementia of the Alzheimer type with depression [see Dementia: B(4) or Major depressive episode: A(2)]

Schizoaffective disorder: A [see Major depressive episode: A(2)]

Schizophrenia: D(9)

Uncomplicated bereavement

blunted affect

Post-traumatic stress disorder: C(6)

Schizoid personality disorder: A(7)

Schizophrenia: D(5)

Schizotypal personality disorder: A(8)

depressed mood

Adjustment disorder with depressed mood

Adjustment disorder with mixed disturbance of emotions and conduct

Adjustment disorder with mixed emotional features

Amphetamine or similarly acting sympatho-mimetic withdrawal: A

Bipolar disorder, depressed: B [see Major depressive episode: A(1)]

Bipolar disorder, mixed: A [see Major depressive episode: A(1)]

Cocaine withdrawal: A

Cyclothymia: A

Dysthymia: A

Hallucinogen hallucinosis: B

Hallucinogen mood disorder: A [see Major depressive episode: A(1)]

Late luteal phase dysphoric disorder: B(4)

Major depression, single or recurrent episode: A [see Major depressive episode: A(1)]

Multi-infarct dementia with depression [see Major depressive episode: A(1)]

Opioid intoxication: B

Organic mood syndrome: A [see Major depressive episode: A(1)]

Phencyclidine (PCP) or similarly acting arylcyclo-hexylamine mood disorder: A [see Major depressive episode: A(1)]

Primary degenerative dementia of the Alzheimer type with depression [see Major depressive episode: A(1)]

Schizoaffective disorder: A [see Major depressive episode: A(1)]

Uncomplicated alcohol withdrawal: A(5)

Uncomplicated bereavement

elevated mood

Bipolar disorder, manic: A [see Manic episode: A]

Bipolar disorder, mixed: A [see Manic episode: A]

Cannabis intoxication: B

Cocaine intoxication: B

Cyclothymia: A [see Hypomanic/Manic episode: A]

Hallucinogen mood disorder: A [see Manic episode: A]

Inhalant intoxication: C(13)

Opioid intoxication: B

Organic mood syndrome: A [see Manic episode: A]

Phencyclidine (PCP) or similarly acting arylcyclo-hexylamine mood disorder: A [see Manic episode: A]

Schizoaffective disorder: A [see Manic episode: A]

flat affect

Schizoaffective disorder: A [see Schizophrenia: A(1)(e)]

Schizophrenia: A(1)(e)

Schizophrenia, disorganized type: B

Schizophreniform disorder: A [see Schizo-phrenia: A(1)(e)]

irritable mood or irritability (in adults)

Alcohol intoxication: B

Amphetamine or similarly acting sympatho-mimetic withdrawal: A

Antisocial personality disorder: C(3)

Bipolar disorder, manic: A [see Manic episode: A]

Bipolar disorder, mixed: A [see Manic episode: A]

Borderline personality disorder: (4)

Cocaine intoxication: B

Cocaine withdrawal: A

Cyclothymia: A [see Hypomanic/Manic episode: A]

Generalized anxiety disorder: D(18)

Hallucinogen mood disorder: A [see Manic episode: A]

Insomnia disorder: B

Late luteal phase dysphoric disorder: B(2)

Nicotine withdrawal: B(2)

Opioid intoxication: B

Organic anxiety syndrome: A [see Generalized anxiety disorder: D(18)]

Organic mood syndrome: A [see Manic episode: A]

Pathological gambling: (4)

Phencyclidine (PCP) or similarly acting arylcyclo-hexylamine mood disorder: A [see Manic episode: A]

Post-traumatic stress disorder: D(2)

Schizoaffective disorder: A [see Manic episode: A]

Sleep-Wake schedule disorder: A [see Insomnia disorder: B]

Uncomplicated alcohol withdrawal: A(5)

Uncomplicated sedative, hypnotic, or anxiolytic withdrawal: A(4)

irritable mood or irritability (in children and adolescents)

Adjustment disorder with depressed mood

Adjustment disorder with mixed disturbance of emotions and conduct

Adjustment disorder with mixed emotional features

Alcohol intoxication: B

Amphetamine or similarly acting sympathomimetic withdrawal: A

Bipolar disorder, depressed: B [see Major depressive episode: A(1)]

Bipolar disorder, manic: A [see Manic episode: A]
Bipolar disorder, mixed: A [see Manic episode: A]
Cocaine intoxication: B
Cocaine withdrawal: A
Cyclothymia: A [see Hypomanic/Manic episode: A]
Dysthymia: A
Generalized anxiety disorder: D(18)
Hallucinogen hallucinosis: B
Hallucinogen mood disorder: A [see Major depressive episode: A(1) or Manic episode: A]
Insomnia disorder: B
Late luteal phase dysphoric disorder: B(2)
Major depression, single or recurrent episode: A [see Major depressive episode: A(1)]
Nicotine withdrawal: B(2)
Opioid intoxication: B
Oppositional defiant disorder: A(6)
Organic anxiety syndrome: A [see Generalized anxiety disorder: D(18)]
Organic mood syndrome: A [see Major depressive episode: A(1) or Manic episode: A]
Pathological gambling: (4)
Phencyclidine (PCP) or similarly acting arylcyclohexylamine mood disorder: A [see Major depressive episode: A(1) or Manic episode: A]
Post-traumatic stress disorder: D(2)
Schizoaffective disorder: A [see Major depressive episode: A(1) or Manic episode: A]
Sleep-Wake schedule disorder: A [see Insomnia disorder: B]
Uncomplicated alcohol withdrawal: A(5)
Uncomplicated bereavement
Uncomplicated sedative, hypnotic, or anxiolytic withdrawal: A(4)

marked mood shifts
    Alcohol intoxication: B
    Borderline personality disorder: (3)
    Brief reactive psychosis: B
    Histrionic personality disorder: (6)
    Late luteal phase dysphoric disorder: B(1)
    Organic personality syndrome: A(1)
    Sedative, hypnotic, or anxiolytic intoxication: B

hallucinations
    Alcohol hallucinosis: A
    Alcohol withdrawal delirium: A [see Delirium: C(2)]
    Amphetamine or similarly acting sympatho-
        mimetic delirium: A [see Delirium: C(2)]
    Bipolar disorder, depressed: B [see Major de-
        pressive episode with psychotic features]
    Bipolar disorder, manic: A [see Manic episode
        with psychotic features]
    Bipolar disorder, mixed: A [see Manic episode
        with psychotic features]
    Brief reactive psychosis: A(3)
    Cocaine delirium: A [see Delirium: C(2)]
    Cocaine intoxication: C(6)
    Delirium: C(2)
    Hallucinogen hallucinosis: C
    Hallucinogen mood disorder: A [see Major de-
        pressive episode with psychotic features or
        Manic episode with psychotic features]
    Major depression, single or recurrent episode: A
        [see Major depressive episode with psy-
        chotic features]
    Multi-infarct dementia with delirium [see Delir-
        ium: C(2)]
    Multi-infarct dementia with depression [see Ma-
        jor depressive episode with psychotic fea-
        tures]

Organic hallucinosis: A

Organic mood syndrome: A [see Major depressive episode with psychotic features or Manic episode with psychotic features]

Phencyclidine (PCP) or similarly acting arylcyclohexylamine delirium: A [see Delirium: C(2)]

Phencyclidine (PCP) or similarly acting arylcyclohexylamine mood disorder: A [see Major depressive episode with psychotic features or Manic episode with psychotic features]

Posthallucinogen perception disorder: A

Primary degenerative dementia of the Alzheimer type with delirium [see Delirium: C(2)]

Primary degenerative dementia of the Alzheimer type with depression [see Major depressive episode with psychotic features]

Schizoaffective disorder: A [see Major depressive episode with psychotic features or Manic episode with psychotic features or Schizophrenia: A(1)(b)]

Schizophrenia: A(1)(b)

Schizophrenia, undifferentiated type: A Schizophreniform disorder: A [see Schizophrenia: A(1)(b)]

Sedative, hypnotic, or anxiolytic withdrawal delirium: A [see Delirium: C(2)]

illusions or perceptual distortions

Alcohol withdrawal delirium: A [see Delirium: C(2)]

Amphetamine or similarly acting sympathomimetic delirium: A [see Delirium: C(2)]

Cocaine delirium: A [see Delirium: C(2)]

Delirium: C(2)

Hallucinogen hallucinosis: C

Multi-infarct dementia with delirium [see Delirium: C(2)]

Phencyclidine (PCP) or similarly acting arylcyclo-
hexylamine delirium: A [see Delirium: C(2)]
Posthallucinogen perception disorder: A
Primary degenerative dementia of the Alzheimer
type with delirium [see Delirium: C(2)]
Schizophrenia: D(8)
Schizotypal personality disorder: A(4)
Sedative, hypnotic, or anxiolytic withdrawal delir-
ium: A [see Delirium: C(2)]

elevated blood pressure
Alcohol withdrawal delirium: B
Amphetamine or similarly acting sympatho-
mimetic intoxication: C(3)
Cocaine intoxication: C(3)
Phencyclidine (PCP) or similarly acting arylcyclo-
hexylamine intoxication: C(2)
Sedative, hypnotic, or anxiolytic withdrawal delir-
ium: B
Uncomplicated alcohol withdrawal: A(3)
Uncomplicated sedative, hypnotic, or anxiolytic
withdrawal: A(3)

pupillary constriction
Opioid intoxication: C

pupillary dilation
Amphetamine or similarly acting sympatho-
mimetic intoxication: C(2)
Cocaine intoxication: C(2)
Hallucinogen hallucinosis: D(1)
Opioid intoxication: C
Opioid withdrawal: A(5)

profuse sweating
Adjustment disorder with physical complaints
Alcohol withdrawal delirium: B

Amphetamine or similarly acting sympathomimetic intoxication: C(4)

Cocaine intoxication: C(4)

Generalized anxiety disorder: D(7)

Hallucinogen hallucinosis: D(3)

Hypochondriasis: A

Late luteal phase dysphoric disorder: B(10)

Opioid withdrawal: A(5)

Organic anxiety syndrome: A [see Generalized
anxiety disorder: D(7) or Panic disorder:
C(5)]

Overanxious disorder: A(4)

Panic disorder: C(5)

Panic disorder with agoraphobia: A [see Panic
disorder: C(5)]

Sedative, hypnotic, or anxiolytic withdrawal delirium: B

Separation anxiety disorder: A(7)

Uncomplicated alcohol withdrawal: A(3)

Uncomplicated sedative, hypnotic, or anxiolytic
withdrawal: A(3)

Undifferentiated somatoform disorder: A

tachycardia

Adjustment disorder with physical complaints

Alcohol withdrawal delirium: B

Amphetamine or similarly acting sympathomimetic intoxication: C(1)

Caffeine intoxication: B(10)

Cannabis intoxication: C(4)

Cocaine intoxication: C(1)

Generalized anxiety disorder: D(6)

Hallucinogen hallucinosis: D(2)

Hypochondriasis: A

Late luteal phase dysphoric disorder: B(10)

Organic anxiety syndrome: A [see Generalized
anxiety disorder: D(6) or Panic disorder:
C(3)]

Panic disorder: C(3)

Panic disorder with agoraphobia: A [see Panic disorder: C(3)]

Phencyclidine (PCP) or similarly acting arylcyclohexylamine intoxication: C(2)

Sedative, hypnotic, or anxiolytic withdrawal delirium: B

Somatization disorder: B(13)

Uncomplicated alcohol withdrawal: A(3)

Uncomplicated sedative, hypnotic, or anxiolytic withdrawal: A(3)

Undifferentiated somatoform disorder: A

chest pain

Adjustment disorder with physical complaints

Hypochondriasis: A

Late luteal phase dysphoric disorder: B(10)

Organic anxiety syndrome: A [see Panic disorder: C(11)]

Overanxious disorder: A(4)

Panic disorder: C(11)

Panic disorder with agoraphobia: A [see Panic disorder: C(11)]

Separation anxiety disorder: A(7)

Somatization disorder: B(14)

Somatoform pain disorder: A

Undifferentiated somatoform disorder: A

abdominal pain

Adjustment disorder with physical complaints

Caffeine intoxication: B(7)

Generalized anxiety disorder: D(10)

Hypochondriasis: A

Late luteal phase dysphoric disorder: B(10)

Organic anxiety syndrome: A [see Generalized anxiety disorder: D(10) or Panic disorder: C(7)]

Overanxious disorder: A(4)

Panic disorder: C(7)

Panic disorder with agoraphobia: A [see Panic disorder: C(7)]

Separation anxiety disorder: A(7)

Somatization disorder: B(2)

Undifferentiated somatoform disorder: A

diarrhea

Adjustment disorder with physical complaints

Caffeine intoxication: B(7)

Generalized anxiety disorder: D(10)

Hypochondriasis: A

Late luteal phase dysphoric disorder: B(10)

Opioid withdrawal: A(6)

Organic anxiety syndrome: A [see Generalized anxiety disorder: D(10) or Panic disorder: C(7)]

Overanxious disorder: A(4)

Panic disorder: C(7)

Panic disorder with agoraphobia: A [see Panic disorder: C(7)]

Separation anxiety disorder: A(7)

Somatization disorder: B(5)

Undifferentiated somatoform disorder: A

vomiting

Adjustment disorder with physical complaints

Amphetamine or similarly acting sympatho-mimetic intoxication: C(5)

Bulimia nervosa: C

Caffeine intoxication: B(7)

Cocaine intoxication: C(5)

Conversion disorder: A

Generalized anxiety disorder: D(10)

Hypochondriasis: A

Late luteal phase dysphoric disorder: B(10)

Opioid withdrawal: A(2)

Organic anxiety syndrome: A [see Generalized anxiety disorder: D(10) or Panic disorder: C(7)]
Overanxious disorder: A(4)
Panic disorder: C(7)
Panic disorder with agoraphobia: A [see Panic disorder: C(7)]
Separation anxiety disorder: A(7)
Somatization disorder: B(1)
Uncomplicated alcohol withdrawal: A(1)
Uncomplicated sedative, hypnotic, or anxiolytic withdrawal: A(1)
Undifferentiated somatoform disorder: A

gait abnormalities
Adjustment disorder with physical complaints
Alcohol intoxication: C(3)
Conversion disorder: A
Inhalant intoxication: C(5)
Multi-infarct dementia: C
Phencyclidine (PCP) or similarly acting arylcyclohexylamine intoxication: C(4)
Sedative, hypnotic, or anxiolytic intoxication: C(3)
Somatization disorder: B(25)
Undifferentiated somatoform disorder: A

nystagmus
Alcohol intoxication: C(4)
Inhalant intoxication: C(2)
Multi-infarct dementia: C
Phencyclidine (PCP) or similarly acting arylcyclohexylamine intoxication: C(1)

paralysis
Adjustment disorder with physical complaints
Conversion disorder: A

Multi-infarct dementia: C
Somatization disorder: B(26)
Undifferentiated somatoform disorder: A

tremor or trembling
Adjustment disorder with physical complaints
Conversion disorder: A
Generalized anxiety disorder: D(1)
Hallucinogen hallucinosis: D(6)
Inhalant intoxication: C(9)
Late luteal phase dysphoric disorder: B(10)
Multi-infarct dementia: C
Organic anxiety syndrome: A [see Generalized
    anxiety disorder: D(1) or Panic disorder:
    C(4)]
Panic disorder: C(4)
Panic disorder with agoraphobia: A [see Panic
    disorder: C(4)]
Uncomplicated alcohol withdrawal: A
Uncomplicated sedative, hypnotic, or anxiolytic
    withdrawal: B(6)
Undifferentiated somatoform disorder: A

physical complaint without organic pathology
Adjustment disorder with physical complaints
Conversion disorder: A
Hypochondriasis: B
Late luteal phase dysphoric disorder: B(10)
Overanxious disorder: A(4)
Separation anxiety disorder: A(7)
Somatization disorder, significance list: (1)
Somatoform pain disorder: B(1)
Undifferentiated somatoform disorder: A

hypersomnia
Adjustment disorder with depressed mood
Alcohol withdrawal delirium: A [see Delirium:
    C(3)]

Amphetamine or similarly acting sympatho-mimetic delirium: A [see Delirium: C(3)]

Amphetamine or similarly acting sympatho-mimetic withdrawal: A(2)

Bipolar disorder, depressed: B [see Major depressive episode: A(4)]

Bipolar disorder, mixed: A [see Major depressive episode: A(4)]

Cocaine delirium: A [see Delirium: C(3)]

Cocaine withdrawal: A(2)

Delirium: C(3)

Dysthymia: B(2)

Hallucinogen mood disorder: A [see Major depressive episode: A(4)]

Hypersomnia disorder: A(1)

Late luteal phase dysphoric disorder: B(9)

Major depression, single or recurrent episode: A [see Major depressive episode: A(4)]

Multi-infarct dementia with delirium [see Delirium: C(3)]

Multi-infarct dementia with depression [see Major depressive episode: A(4)]

Organic mood syndrome: A [see Major depressive episode: A(4)]

Phencyclidine (PCP) or similarly acting arylcyclo-hexylamine delirium: A [see Delirium: C(3)]

Phencyclidine (PCP) or similarly acting arylcyclo-hexylamine mood disorder: A [see Major depressive episode: A(4)]

Primary degenerative dementia of the Alzheimer type with delirium [see Delirium: C(3)]

Primary degenerative dementia of the Alzheimer type with depression [see Major depressive episode: A(4)]

Schizoaffective disorder: A [see Major depressive episode: A(4)]

Sedative, hypnotic, or anxiolytic withdrawal delirium: A [see Delirium: C(3)]

Sleep-Wake schedule disorder: A [see Hypersomnia disorder: A(1)]
Uncomplicated bereavement

insomnia
Adjustment disorder with depressed mood
Alcohol withdrawal delirium: A [see Delirium: C(3)]
Amphetamine or similarly acting sympathomimetic delirium: A [see Delirium: C(3)]
Amphetamine or similarly acting sympathomimetic withdrawal: A(2)
Bipolar disorder, depressed: B [see Major depressive episode: A(4)]
Bipolar disorder, manic: A [see Manic episode: B(2)]
Bipolar disorder, mixed: A [see Manic episode: B(2)]
Caffeine intoxication: B(4)
Cocaine delirium: A [see Delirium: C(3)]
Cocaine withdrawal: A(2)
Cyclothymia: A [see Hypomanic/Manic episode: B(2)]
Delirium: C(3)
Dysthymia: B(2)
Generalized anxiety disorder: D(17)
Hallucinogen mood disorder: A [see Major depressive episode: A(4) or Manic episode: B(2)]
Insomnia disorder: A
Late luteal phase dysphoric disorder: B(9)
Major depression, single or recurrent episode: A [see Major depressive episode: A(4)]
Multi-infarct dementia with delirium [see Delirium: C(3)]
Multi-infarct dementia with depression [see Major depressive episode: A(4)]
Opioid withdrawal: A(9)

Organic anxiety syndrome: A [see Generalized anxiety disorder: D(17)]

Organic mood syndrome: A [see Major depressive episode: A(4) or Manic episode: B(2)]

Phencyclidine (PCP) or similarly acting arylcyclohexylamine delirium: A [see Delirium: C(3)]

Phencyclidine (PCP) or similarly acting arylcyclohexylamine mood disorder: A [see Major depressive episode: A(4) or Manic episode: B(2)]

Post-traumatic stress disorder: D(1)

Primary degenerative dementia of the Alzheimer type with delirium [see Delirium: C(3)]

Primary degenerative dementia of the Alzheimer type with depression [see Major depressive episode: A(4)]

Schizoaffective disorder: A [see Major depressive episode: A(4) or Manic episode: B(2)]

Sedative, hypnotic, or anxiolytic withdrawal delirium: A [see Delirium: C(3)]

Sleep-Wake schedule disorder: A [see Insomnia disorder: A]

Uncomplicated bereavement

Uncomplicated sedative, hypnotic, or anxiolytic withdrawal: A(7)

bizarre delusions

Bipolar disorder, depressed: B [see Major depressive episode with psychotic features]

Bipolar disorder, manic: A [see Manic episode with psychotic features]

Bipolar disorder, mixed: A [see Manic episode with psychotic features]

Brief reactive psychosis: A(2)

Cannabis delusional disorder: A

Hallucinogen delusional disorder: A

Hallucinogen mood disorder: A [see Major de-

pressive episode with psychotic features or
       Manic episode with psychotic features]
Induced psychotic disorder: A
Major depression, single or recurrent episode: A
       [see Major depressive episode with psy-
       chotic features]
Multi-infarct dementia with delusions
Multi-infarct dementia with depression [see Ma-
       jor depressive episodewith psychotic fea-
       tures]
Organic delusional syndrome: A
Organic mood syndrome: A [see Major de-
       pressive episode with psychotic features or
       Manic episode with psychotic features]
Phencyclidine (PCP) or similarly acting arylcyclo-
       hexylamine delusional disorder: A
Phencyclidine (PCP) or similarly acting arylcyclo-
       hexylamine mood disorder: A [see Major de-
       pressive episode with psychotic features or
       Manic episode with psychotic features]
Primary degenerative dementia of the Alzheimer
       type with delusions
Primary degenerative dementia of the Alzheimer
       type with depression [see Major depressive
       episode with psychotic features]
Schizoaffective disorder: A [see Major depressive
       episode with psychotic features or Manic
       episode with psychotic features or Schizo-
       phrenia: A(2)]
Schizophrenia: A(2)
Schizophrenia, undifferentiated type: A
Schizophreniform disorder: A [see Schizo-
       phrenia: A(2)]

nonbizarre delusions
       Bipolar disorder, depressed: B [see Major de-
              pressive episode with psychotic features]
       Bipolar disorder, manic: A [see Manic episode

with psychotic features]

Bipolar disorder, mixed: A [see Manic episode with psychotic features]

Brief reactive psychosis: A(2)

Cannabis delusional disorder: A

Delusional disorder: A

Hallucinogen delusional disorder: A

Hallucinogen mood disorder: A [see Major depressive episode with psychotic features or Manic episode with psychotic features]

Induced psychotic disorder: A

Major depression, single or recurrent episode: A [see Major depressive episode with psychotic features]

Multi-infarct dementia with delusions

Multi-infarct dementia with depression [see Major depressive episode with psychotic features]

Organic delusional syndrome: A

Organic mood syndrome: A [see Major depressive episode with psychotic features or Manic episode with psychotic features]

Phencyclidine (PCP) or similarly acting arylcyclohexylamine delusional disorder: A

Phencyclidine (PCP) or similarly acting arylcyclohexylamine mood disorder: A [see Major depressive episode with psychotic features or Manic episode with psychotic features]

Primary degenerative dementia of the Alzheimer type with delusions

Primary degenerative dementia of the Alzheimer type with depression [see Major depressive episode with psychotic features]

Schizoaffective disorder: A [see Major depressive episode with psychotic features or Manic episode with psychotic features or Schizophrenia A(1)(a)]

Schizophrenia: A(1)(a)

Schizophrenia, undifferentiated type: A
Schizophreniform disorder: A [see Schizo-
    phrenia: A(1)(a)]

grandiosity
    Amphetamine or similarly acting sympatho-
        mimetic intoxication: B
    Bipolar disorder, manic: A [see Manic episode:
        B(1)]
    Bipolar disorder, mixed: A [see Manic episode:
        B(1)]
    Cocaine intoxication: B
    Cyclothymia: A [see Hypomanic/Manic episode:
        B(1)]
    Hallucinogen mood disorder: A [see Manic epi-
        sode: B(1)]
    Narcissistic personality disorder: (3)
    Organic mood syndrome: A [see Manic episode:
        B(1)]
    Phencyclidine (PCP) or similarly acting arylcyclo-
        hexylamine mood disorder: A [see Manic
        episode: B(1)]
    Schizoaffective disorder: A [see Manic episode:
        B(1)]

feelings of hopelessness
    Adjustment disorder with depressed mood
    Adjustment disorder with mixed disturbance of
        emotions and conduct
    Adjustment disorder with mixed emotional fea-
        tures
    Amphetamine or similarly acting sympatho-
        mimetic withdrawal: A
    Bipolar disorder, depressed: B [see Major de-
        pressive episode: A(1)]
    Bipolar disorder, mixed: A [see Major depressive
        episode: A(1)]
    Cocaine withdrawal: A

Cyclothymia: A
Dysthymia: B(6)
Hallucinogen hallucinosis: B
Hallucinogen mood disorder: A [see Major depressive episode: A(1)]
Late luteal phase dysphoric disorder: B(4)
Major depression, single or recurrent episode: A [see Major depressive episode: A(1)]
Multi-infarct dementia with depression [see Major depressive episode: A(1)]
Opioid intoxication: B
Organic mood syndrome: A [see Major depressive episode: A(1)]
Phencyclidine (PCP) or similarly acting arylcyclohexylamine mood disorder: A [see Major depressive episode: A(1)]
Primary degenerative dementia of the Alzheimer type with depression [see Major depressive episode: A(1)]
Schizoaffective disorder: A [see Major depressive episode: A(1)]
Uncomplicated alcohol withdrawal: A(5)
Uncomplicated bereavement

ideas of reference
Hallucinogen hallucinosis: B
Schizophrenia: D(7)
Schizotypal personality disorder: A(1)

paranoid ideation (nondelusional)
Amphetamine or similarly acting sympathomimetic intoxication: B
Cannabis intoxication: B
Cocaine intoxication: B
Hallucinogen hallucinosis: B
Organic personality syndrome: A(5)
Paranoid personality disorder: A(3)
Schizotypal personality disorder: A(9)

suicidal ideation

Bipolar disorder, depressed: B [see Major depressive episode: A(9)]

Bipolar disorder, mixed: A [see Major depressive episode: A(9)]

Borderline personality disorder: (5)

Hallucinogen mood disorder: A [see Major depressive episode: A(9)]

Major depression, single or recurrent episode: A [see Major depressive episode: A(9)]

Multi-infarct dementia with depression [see Major depressive episode: A(9)]

Organic mood syndrome: A [see Major depressive episode: A(9)]

Phencyclidine (PCP) or similarly acting arylcyclohexylamine mood disorder: A [see Major depressive episode: A(9)]

Primary degenerative dementia of the Alzheimer type with depression [see Major depressive episode: A(9)]

Schizoaffective disorder: A [see Major depressive episode: A(9)]

Diagnostic Index:
Index of DSM-III-R Diagnoses
and Selected Diagnostic Terms

Abuse 109
  Alcohol 109
  Amphetamine or similarly acting sympathomimetic 110
  Cannabis 110
  Cocaine 110
  Hallucinogen 110
  Inhalant 110
  Opioid 110
  Phencyclidine (PCP) or similarly acting arylcyclohexylamine 110
  Psychoactive substance 110
  Psychoactive substance, not otherwise specified 111
  Sedative, hypnotic, or anxiolytic 110
Academic or work inhibition. *See* Adjustment disorder with work (or academic) inhibition 185
Academic problem 203
Academic skills disorders 52
  Developmental arithmetic disorder 52
  Developmental expressive writing disorder 52
  Developmental reading disorder 53
Acrophobia. *See* Simple phobia 144
Acute
  confusional state. *See* Delirium 77

   paranoid disorder. *See* Psychotic disorder not
      otherwise specified 124
   schizophrenic episode. *See* Brief reactive psycho-
      sis 121 or Schizophreniform disorder 122
Additional codes 209
   Diagnosis or condition deferred on Axis I 209
   Diagnosis or condition deferred on Axis II 210
   No diagnosis or condition on Axis I 209
   No diagnosis or condition on Axis II 210
   Unspecified mental disorder (nonpsychotic) 209
Adjustment disorder 183
   not otherwise specified 185
   with anxious mood 184
   with atypical features. *See* Adjustment disorder
      not otherwise specified 185
   with depressed mood 184
   with disturbance of conduct 184
   with mixed disturbance of emotions and con-
      duct 184
   with mixed emotional features 184
   with physical complaints 185
   with withdrawal 185
   with work (or academic) inhibition 185
Adjustment reaction. *See* Adjustment disorder 183
Adolescence
   Avoidant disorder of childhood or 62
   Disorders usually first evident in infancy, child-
      hood, or 47
   Gender identity disorder of, or adulthood 67
Adolescent antisocial behavior. *See* Childhood or
   adolescent antisocial behavior 204
Adult antisocial behavior 204
Affective disorders. *See* Mood disorders 125
Agoraphobia
   with panic attacks. *See* Panic Disorder with agora-
      phobia 140
   without history of panic disorder 142

without panic attacks. *See* Agoraphobia without
    history of panic disorder   142
Alcohol use disorders, abuse/dependence   109
Alcohol-induced organic mental disorders   86
    amnestic disorder   88
    dementia. *See* Dementia associated with alco-
        holism   88
    hallucinosis   88
    idiosyncratic intoxication   87
    intoxication   86
    jealousy. *See* Delusional (paranoid) disorder, jeal-
        ous type   120
    withdrawal delirium   88
    withdrawal, Uncomplicated   87
Alzheimer's disease. *See* Primary degenerative de-
    mentia of the Alzheimer type   84
Amnesia
    anterograde. *See* Amnestic syndrome   80 or Psy-
        chogenic amnesia   157
    Psychogenic   157
    retrograde. *See* Amnestic syndrome   80 or Psy-
        chogenic amnesia   157
Amnestic disorder
    Alcohol   88
    associated with Axis III physical disorders or
        conditions or is unknown   105
    Other or unspecified psychoactive substance   104
    Sedative, hypnotic, or anxiolytic   103
Amnestic syndrome   80
Amphetamine or similarly acting sympathomimetic
    use disorders, abuse/dependence   109
Amphetamine- or similarly acting sympathomimetic-
    induced organic mental disorders   89
    delirium   90
    delusional disorder   90
    intoxication   89
    withdrawal   89

Anankastic personality. *See* Obsessive compulsive personality disorder 199

Anorexia nervosa 63

Antisocial
  behavior, adult 204
  behavior, childhood and adolescent 204
  personality disorder 193

Anxiety disorders (or anxiety and phobic neuroses) 142
  Agoraphobia without history of panic disorder 148
  Generalized anxiety disorder 150
  not otherwise specified 150
  Obsessive compulsive disorder 145
  Panic disorder 139
  Panic disorder with agoraphobia 140
  Panic disorder without agoraphobia 142
  Post-traumatic stress disorder 146
  Simple phobia 144
  Social phobia 143

Anxiety disorders of childhood or adolescence 61
  Avoidant disorder of childhood or adolescence 62
  Overanxious disorder 62
  Separation anxiety disorder 61

Anxiety neuroses. *See* Panic disorder 139 or Generalized anxiety disorder 148

Anxious mood. *See* Adjustment disorder with anxious mood 184

Arithmetic disorder. *See* Developmental arithmetic disorder 52

Arousal, sexual. *See* Female sexual arousal disorder 165 or Male erectile disorder 166

Arteriosclerotic dementia. *See* Multi-infarct dementia 85

Articulation disorder. *See* Developmental articulation disorder 53

Arylcyclohexylamine. *See* Phencyclidine (PCP) or similarly acting arylcyclohexylamine

Asthenic personality. *See* Dependent personality disorder   198

Attention deficit disorder
  with hyperactivity. *See* Attention-deficit hyperactivity disorder   56
  without hyperactivity. *See* Undifferentiated attention-deficit disorder   74

Attention-deficit
  hyperactivity disorder   56
  Undifferentiated, disorder   74

Atypical
  affective disorder. *See* Bipolar disorder not otherwise specified   134 or Depressive disorder not otherwise specified   137
  anxiety disorder. *See* Anxiety disorder not otherwise specified   150
  bipolar disorder. *See* Bipolar disorder not otherwise specified   134
  depression. *See* Depressive disorder not otherwise specified   137
  development. *See* Pervasive development disorders   49
  dissociative disorder. *See* Disssociative disorder not otherwise specified   158
  eating disorder. *See* Eating disorder not otherwise specified   65
  factitious disorder with physical symptoms. *See* Factitious disorder not otherwise specified   178
  features, Adjustment disorder with. *See* Adjustment disorder not otherwise specified   185
  gender identity disorder. *See* Gender disorder not otherwise specified   68
  impulse control disorder. *See* Impulse control disorder not otherwise specified   181
  mixed or other personality disorder. *See* Personality disorder not otherwise specified   200

or mixed organic brain syndrome. See Organic Mental Syndrome not otherwise specified 84

paranoid disorder. See Psychotic disorder not otherwise specified 124

paraphilia. See Paraphilia not otherwise specified 164

pervasive developmental disorder. See Pervasive developmental disorder not otherwise specified 52

psychosexual dysfunction. See Sexual dysfunction not otherwise specified 168

psychosis. See Psychotic disorder not otherwise specified 124

somatoform disorder. See Undifferentiated somatoform disorder 155 or Somatoform disorder not otherwise specified 156

specific developmental disorder. See Specific developmental disorder not otherwise specified 55

stereotyped movement disorder. See Tic disorder not otherwise specified 70 or Stereotypy/habit disorder 74

tic disorder. See Tic disorder not otherwise specified 70

Autism, Infantile. See Autistic disorder 49

Autistic disorder 49

Avoidant
  disorder of childhood or adolescence 62
  personality disorder 147

Barbiturate. See Sedative, hypnotic or anxiolytic

Behavior disorders. See Disruptive behavior disorders 56

Bereavement, Uncomplicated, 208

Bipolar II. See Bipolar disorder not otherwise specified 134

Bipolar disorder   132
  depressed   133
  manic   133
  mixed   132
  not otherwise specified   134
Blood-injury phobia. *See* Simple phobia   144
Body dysmorphic disorder   151
Borderline
  intellectual functioning   204
  mental retardation. *See* Borderline intellectual
    functioning   204
  personality disorder   196
  schizophrenia. *See* Schizotypal personality disor-
    der   191
Brief reactive psychosis   121
Briquet's syndrome. *See* Somatization disorder   153
Bulimia nervosa   64

Caffeine-induced organic mental disorder   91
  Caffeine intoxication   91
Caffeinism. *See* Caffeine intoxication   91
Cannabis use disorders, abuse/dependence   110
Cannabis-induced organic mental disorders   91
  delusional disorder   92
  hallucinosis. *See* Cannabis intoxication   91
  intoxication   91
Cardiac neurosis. *See* Hypochondriasis   152
Catatonic type, Schizophrenia   117
Child abuse. *See* Parent-child problem   207
Childhood, Gender identity disorder of   65
Childhood or adolescence
  Anxiety disorders of   61
  Avoidant disorder of   62
  Disorders usually first evident in infancy   47
Childhood onset pervasive developmental disorder.
    See Autistic disorder   49

Childhood or adolescent antisocial behavior 204
Childhood psychosis. *See* Pervasive developmental disorders 49
Childhood, Reactive attachment disorder. *See* Reactive attachment disorder of infancy or early childhood 73
Childhood schizophrenia. *See* Pervasive developmental disorders 49
Chronic mood disorders
  Cyclothymia 133
  Dysthymia 136
Chronic motor or vocal tic disorder 69
Claustrophobia. *See* Simple phobia 144
Cluttering 72
Cocaine use disorders, abuse/dependence 110
Cocaine-induced organic mental disorders 92
  delirium 93
  delusional disorder 94
  intoxication 92
  withdrawal 93
Compensation neurosis. *See* Psychological factors affecting physical condition 187
Compulsions. *See* Obsessive compulsive disorder 145
Compulsive personality. *See* Obsessive compulsive personality disorder 199
Concentration camp syndrome. *See* Post-traumatic stress disorder 146
Conduct disorder 58
  atypical. *See* Conduct disorder, undifferentiated type 59
  group type 59
  socialized, nonaggressive. *See* Conduct disorder, group type 59
  solitary aggressive type 59
  undersocialized, aggressive. *See* Conduct disorder, solitary aggressive type 59

undersocialized, nonagressive. *See* Conduct disorder, undifferentiated type   59
  undifferentiated type   59
Conduct disturbance. *See* Adjustment disorder with disturbance of conduct   184
Conjugal paranoia. *See* Delusional (paranoid) disorder, jealous type   120
Conversion disorder   151
Coordination disorder. *See* Developmental coordination disorder   55
Coprophilia. *See* Paraphilia not otherwise specified   164
Crack. *See* Cocaine
Cyclothymia   133
Cyclothymic disorder. *See* Cyclothymia   133
Cyclothymic personality. *See* Cyclothymia   133

Deferred diagnoses
  Diagnosis or condition deferred on Axis I   209
  Diagnosis or condition deferred on Axis II   210
Delirium   77
  Alcohol withdrawal   88
  Amphetamine or similarly acting sympathomimetic   90
  associated with axis III physical disorders or conditions, or whose etiology is unknown   105
  Cocaine   93
  Multi-infarct dementia, with   85
  Other or unspecified psychoactive substance   104
  Phencyclidine (PCP) or similarly acting arylcyclohexylamine   99
  Primary degenerative dementia of the Alzheimer type, presenile onset, with   85
  Primary degenerative dementia of the Alzheimer type, senile onset, with   84
  Sedative, hypnotic, or anxiolytic withdrawal   102
  tremens. *See* Alcohol withdrawal delirium   88

Delusional (paranoid) disorder   119
  erotomanic type   120
  grandiose type   120
  jealous type   120
  persecutory type   120
  somatic type   120
  unspecified type   120
Delusional disorder
  Amphetamine or similarly acting sym-
    pathomimetic   90
  Cocaine   94
  Hallucinogen   95
  Organic, associated with axis III physical disorders
    or conditions, or whose etiology is un-
    known   105
  Other or unspecified psychoactive substance   104
  Phencyclidine (PCP) or similarly acting
    arylcyclohexylamine   100
Delusions
  Multi-infarct dementia, with   85
  Primary degenerative dementia of the Alzheimer
    type, presenile onset, with   85
  Primary degenerative dementia of the Alzheimer
    type, senile onset, with   84
  Dementia   78
  associated with alcoholism   88
  associated with axis III physical disorders or con-
    ditions, or whose etiology is unknown   105
  Multi-infarct   85
  Other or unspecified psychoactive substance   104
  Presenile, not otherwise specified   86
  Primary degenerative, of the Alzheimer type   84
  Senile, not otherwise specified   86
Dementias arising in the senium and presenium   84
  Multi-infarct dementia   85
  Presenile dementia not otherwise specified   86
  Primary degenerative dementia of the Alzheimer
    type, presenile onset   85

Primary degenerative dementia of the Alzheimer type, senile onset   84
Senile dementia not otherwise specified   86
Dependence   107
  Alcohol   109
  Amphetamine or similarly acting sym-pathomimetic   109
  Cannabis   110
  Cocaine   110
  Hallucinogen   110
  Inhalant   110
  Nicotine   110
  on combination of opioid and other nonalcoholic substances. *See* Polysubstance dependence   110
  on combination of substances, excluding opioids and alcohol. *See* Polysubstance dependence   110
  Opioid   110
  Phencyclidine (PCP) or similarly acting arylcyclo-hexylamine   110
  Polysubstance   110
  Psychoactive substance   107
  Psychoactive substance, not otherwise spec-ified   111
  Sedative, hypnotic, or anxiolytic   110
Dependent personality disorder   198
Depersonalization disorder   158
Depersonalization neurosis. *See* Depersonalization disorder   158
Depressed mood. *See* Adjustment disorder with depressed mood   184
Depressive disorders   135
  Depressive neurosis. *See* Dysthymia   136
  Dysthymia   136
  Major depression, single episode or recur-rent   135
  not otherwise specified   137

Depressive episode, Major   128
Derealization. *See* Depersonalization disorder   158
Developmental disorders   47
  Autistic disorder   49
  Developmental arithmetic disorder   52
  Developmental articulation disorder   53
  Developmental coordination disorder   55
  Developmental expressive language disorder   54
  Developmental expressive writing disorder   52
  Developmental language disorder. *See* Develop-
    mental expressive language disorder   54 or De-
    velopmental receptive language disorder   54
  Developmental reading disorder   53
  Developmental receptive language disorder   54
  Language and speech disorders   53
  Mental retardation   47
  Motor skills disorders   55
  Pervasive developmental disorder not otherwise
    specified   52
  Pervasive developmental disorders   49
  not otherwise specified   56
  Specific developmental disorder not otherwise
    specified   55
  Specific developmental disorders   52
Deviation, Sexual. *See* Paraphilias   161
Diagnosis or condition deferred on Axis I   209
Diagnosis or condition deferred on Axis II   210
Disintegrative psychosis. *See* Pervasive developmen-
  tal disorders   49
Disorganized type, Schizophrenia   117
Disruptive behavior disorders   56
  Attention-deficit hyperactivity disorder   56
  Conduct disorder   58
  Oppositional defiant disorder   60
Dissociative disorders   157
  Depersonalization disorder   158
  Depersonalization neurosis. *See* Depersonaliza-
    tion disorder   158

Multiple personality disorder   157
not otherwise specified   158
Psychogenic amnesia   157
Psychogenic fugue   157
Dream anxiety disorder (Nightmare disorder)   175
Dyslexia. *See* Developmental reading disorder   53
Dysmorphophobia. *See* Body dysmorphic disorder   151
Dyspareunia   167
Dyssomnias   171
Hypersomnia disorders   172
Insomnia disorders   171
not otherwise specified   174
Sleep-wake schedule disorder   174
Dysthymia   136
Dysthymic disorder. *See* Dysthymia   136

Eating Disorders   63
Anorexia nervosa   63
Bulimia nervosa   64
not otherwise specified   65
Pica   64
Rumination disorder of infancy   65
Ego-dystonic homosexuality. *See* Sexual disorder not otherwise specified   168
Ejaculation, Premature   167
Elective mutism   72
Elimination disorders   70
Functional encopresis   70
Functional enuresis   71
Encopresis, Functional   70
Enuresis, Functional   71
Erectile dysfunction. *See* Male erectile disorder   166
Erotomanic type, Delusional (paranoid) disorder   120
Exhibitionism   161
Explosive disorder, Intermittent,   179

Expressive
   language disorder. *See* Developmental expressive
      language disorder   54
   writing disorder. *See* Developmental expressive
      writing disorder   52

Factitious disorders   177
   not otherwise specified   178
   with physical symptoms   177
   with psychological symptoms   177
Failure to thrive. *See* Reactive attachment disorder
   of infancy or early childhood   73
Family circumstances, Other specified   207
Female sexual arousal disorder   165
Fetishism   161
Flashbacks. *See* Posthallucinogen perception disorder   95
Folie à deux. *See* Induced psychotic disorder   123
Frigidity. *See* Hypoactive sexual desire disorder   165, Female sexual arousal disorder   165,
   or Inhibited female orgasm   166
Frotteurism   162
Fugue state. *See* Psychogenic fugue   157
Functional
   dyspareunia. *See* Dyspareunia   167
   encopresis   70
   enuresis   71
   vaginismus. *See* Vaginismus   168

Gambling. *See* Pathological gambling   179
Ganser's syndrome. *See* Dissociative disorder not
   otherwise specified   158
Gender identity disorders   65
   not otherwise specified   68
   of adolescence or adulthood, nontranssexual type
      (GIDAANT)   67
   of childhood   65
   Transsexualism   67

Generalized anxiety disorder 148
Gilles de la Tourette's syndrome. *See* Tourette's
    disorder 69
Grandiose type, Delusional (paranoid) disorder 120
Group type, Conduct disorder 59

Hallucinogen use disorders, abuse/depen-
    dence 110
Hallucinogen-induced organic mental disorders 94
    affective disorder. *See* Hallucinogen mood disor-
        der 95
    delusional disorder 95
    hallucinosis 94
    mood disorder 95
    Posthallucinogen perception disorder 95
Hallucinosis
    Alcohol 88
    Hallucinogen 94
    Organic, associated with axis III disorders or
        conditions, or whose etiology is unknown 105
    Other or unspecific psychoactive substance 104
Hebephrenic schizophrenia. *See* Schizophrenia, dis-
    organized type 118
Heller's syndrome. *See* Pervasive developmental dis-
    orders 49
Histrionic personality disorder 192
Homosexuality, Ego-dystonic. *See* Sexual disorder
    not otherwise specified 168
Hospitalism. *See* Reactive attachment disorder of
    infancy or early childhood 73
Hyperactive child syndrome. *See* Attention-deficit
    hyperactivity disorder 56
Hyperactivity, Attention-deficit, disorder 56
Hyperkinesis with developmental delay. *See* Atten-
    tion-deficit hyperactivity disorder 56
Hypersomnia disorders 172
    Primary 173
    related to a known organic factor 173

related to another mental disorder (non-
    organic) 173
Hypnotic. *See* Sedative, hypnotic, or anxiolytic
Hypoactive sexual desire disorder 165
Hypochondriacal neurosis. *See* Hypochondriasis 152
Hypochondriasis 152
Hypomanic disorder. *See* Bipolar disorder not other-
    wise specified 134
Hypomanic episode. *See* Manic episode 125
Hypoxyphilia. *See* Sexual masochism 163
Hysterical neurosis
    conversion type. *See* Conversion disorder 151
    dissociative type. *See* Dissociative disorders 157
Hysterical personality. *See* Histrionic personality dis-
    order 192
Hysterical psychosis. *See* Brief reactive psycho-
    sis 121 or Factitious disorder with psychologi-
    cal symptoms 177

Identity disorder 72
Identity disorders, Gender 65
Immature personality. *See* Personality disorder not
    otherwise specified 200
Impulse control disorders not elsewhere classi-
    fied 179
    Intermittent explosive disorder 179
    Kleptomania 179
    Pathological gambling 180
    Pyromania 180
    Trichotillomania 181
Impulse control disorder not otherwise spec-
    ified 181
Impulsive personality. *See* Personality disorder not
    otherwise specified 200
Induced psychotic disorder 123
Infancy, childhood, or adolescence, Disorders of.
    See Disorders usually first evident in infancy,
    childhood, or adolescence 47

Infancy, Reactive attachment disorder. *See* Reactive attachment disorder of infancy or early childhood   73

Infancy, Rumination disorder of   65

Infantile autism. *See* Autistic disorder   49

Inhalant use disorders, abuse/dependence   110

Inhalant-induced organic mental disorder   96
  intoxication   96

Inhibited
  female orgasm   166
  male orgasm   167
  sexual desire. *See* Hypoactive sexual desire disorder   165 or Sexual aversion disorder   165
  sexual excitement. *See* Female sexual arousal disorder   165 or Male erectile disorder   166

Insomnia disorders   171
  Primary   172
  related to a known organic factor   172
  related to another mental disorder (non-organic)   171

Interpersonal problem, Other   207

Intermittent explosive disorder   179

Intoxication   83
  Alcohol   86
  Alcohol idiosyncratic   87
  Amphetamine or similarly acting sympathomimetic   89
  Caffeine   91
  Cocaine   92
  Hallucinogen. *See* Hallucinogen hallucinosis   94
  Inhalant   96
  Opioid   97
  Other or unspecified substance   103
  Phencyclidine (PCP) or similarly acting arylcyclohexylamine   98
  Sedative, hypnotic, or anxiolytic   101

Involutional melancholia. *See* Major depressive episode, melancholic type   131

Isolated explosive disorder. *See* Impulse control disorder not otherwise specified 181

Jealous type, Delusional (paranoid) disorder 120

Kanner's syndrome. *See* Autistic disorder 49
Kleptomania 179
Klismaphilia. *See* Paraphilia not otherwise specified 164
Korsakoff's syndrome. *See* Alcohol amnestic disorder 88

LSD. *See* Hallucinogen
Labile personality disorder. *See* Cyclothymia 133
Language and speech disorders (developmental) 53
Developmental articulation disorder 53
Developmental expressive language disorder 54
Developmental receptive language disorder 54
Late luteal phase dysphoric disorder 213
Latent schizophrenia. *See* Schizotypal personality disorder 191

Major affective disorders. *See* Bipolar disorder 132 or Major depression 135
Major depression, single episode or recurrent 135
Major depressive episode 128
Male erectile disorder 166
Malingering 205
Manic-depression. *See* Bipolar disorder 132
Manic episode 125
Marijuana. *See* Cannabis
Marital problem 206
Masochism, Sexual 163
Masochistic personality. *See* Self-defeating personality disorder 216
Melancholia. *See* Major depressive episode, melancholic type 131

Mental retardation   47
  Mild   48
  Moderate   48
  Profound   48
  Severe   48
  Unspecified   48
Mild mental retardation   48
Minimal brain dysfunction. *See* Attention-deficit hy-
    peractivity disorder   56
Mixed, Bipolar disorder   132
Mixed disturbance of emotions and conduct. *See*
    Adjustment disorder with mixed disturbance of
    emotions and conduct   184
Mixed emotional features. *See* Adjustment disorder
    with mixed emotional features   184
Mixed or other personality disorder, Atypical. *See*
    Personality disorder not otherwise spec-
    ified   200
Mixed or unspecified substance abuse, Other. *See*
    Psychoactive substance abuse not otherwise
    specified   111
Mixed or unspecified substance-induced mental dis-
    order. *See* Other or unspecified psychoactive
    substance organic mental disorder not other-
    wise specified   104
Mixed specific developmental disorder. *See* Specific
    developmental disorders   52
Moderate mental retardation   48
Mood disorders   125
  Bipolar disorder   132
  Bipolar disorder not otherwise specified   134
  Cyclothymia   133
  Depressive disorder not otherwise specified   137
  Dysthymia   136
  Major depression, single episode or recur-
    rent   135
  Seasonal pattern   131

Motor, chronic, or vocal tic disorder. _See_ Chronic
    motor or vocal tic disorder   69
Motor skills disorder   55
  Developmental coordination disorder   55
Movement disorders. _See_ Tic disorders   68 or
    Stereotypy/habit disorder   74
Multi-infarct dementia   85
Multiple personality disorder   157
Munchausen syndrome. _See_ Factitious disorder with
    physical symptoms   177
Mutism, Elective   72

Narcissistic personality disorder   192
Necrophilia. _See_ Paraphilia not otherwise spec-
    ified   164
Neurasthenia. _See_ Dysthymia   136
Neurosis
  Anxiety. _See_ Panic disorder   139 or Generalized
    anxiety disorder   148
  Depersonalization. _See_ Depersonalization disor-
    der   158
  Depressive. _See_ Dysthymia   136, Major depres-
    sion   135, or Adjustment disorder with de-
    pressed mood   184
  Hypochondriacal. _See_ Hypochondriasis   152
  Hysterical, conversion type. _See_ Conversion disor-
    der   151 or Somatoform pain disorder   155
  Hysterical, dissociative type. _See_ Dissociative dis-
    orders   157 or Sleepwalking disorder   176
  Neurasthenic. _See_ Dysthymia   136
  Obsessive compulsive. _See_ Obsessive compulsive
    disorder   145
  Phobic. _See_ Simple phobia   144, Social pho-
    bia   143, or Separation anxiety disorder   61
Nicotine dependence   110
Nicotine-induced organic mental disorder   97
  withdrawal   97

Nightmare disorder. *See* Dream anxiety disorder 175
No diagnosis or condition on Axis I 209
No diagnosis or condition on Axis II 210
Noncompliance with medical treatment 206
Nonpsychotic mental disorder. *See* Unspecified mental disorder (nonpsychotic) 209

Obsessive compulsive disorder 145
Obsessive compulsive personality disorder 199
Occupational problem 206
Opioid use disorders, abuse/dependence 110
Opioid-induced organic mental disorders 97
  intoxication 97
  withdrawal 98
Oppositional defiant disorder 60
Organic affective syndrome. *See* Organic mood syndrome 81
Organic anxiety
  disorder 105
  syndrome 82
Organic brain syndromes. *See* Organic mental syndromes 77
Organic delusional
  disorder 105
  syndrome 81
Organic hallucinosis 81
  associated with axis III disorders or conditions, or whose etiology is unknown 105
Organic mental disorders 84
  associated with Axis III physical disorders or conditions, or whose etiology in unknown 105
  Dementias arising in the senium and presenium 84
  not otherwise specified 105
  Psychoactive substance-induced 103
Organic mental syndromes 77

Amnestic syndrome   80
Delirium   77
Dementia   78
Intoxication   83
Organic affective syndrome. *See* Organic mood
   syndrome   81
Organic anxiety syndrome   82
Organic delusional syndrome   81
Organic hallucinosis   81
Organic mood syndrome   81
Organic personality syndrome   82
not otherwise specified   84
Withdrawal   83
Organic mood
   disorder   105
   syndrome   81
Organic personality
   disorder   105
   syndrome   82
Orgasm disorders   166
   Inhibited female orgasm   166
   Inhibited male orgasm   167
   Premature ejaculation   167
Other developmental disorders   56
   Developmental disorder not otherwise spec-
      ified   56
Other disorders of infancy, childhood, or adoles-
      cence   72
   Elective mutism   72
   Identity disorder   72
   Reactive attachment disorder of infancy or early
      childhood   73
   Stereotypy/habit disorder   74
   Undifferentiated attention-deficit disorder   74
Other or unspecified psychoactive substance-in-
      duced organic mental disorders   104
Other interpersonal problem   207

Other, mixed or unspecified substance abuse. *See* Psychoactive substance abuse not otherwise specified 111

Other psychosexual disorders. *See* Sexual disorder not otherwise specified 168

Other sexual disorders 168
Sexual disorder not otherwise specified 168

Other specified family circumstances 207

Other specified substance dependence. *See* Psychoactive substance dependence not otherwise specified 111

Overanxious disorder 62

Pain, Somatoform. *See* Somatoform pain disorder 155

Panic disorder 139
with agoraphobia 140
without agoraphobia 142

Paranoia. *See* Delusional (paranoid) disorder 119

Paranoid disorder. *See* Delusional (paranoid) disorder 119
Acute. *See* Psychotic disorder not otherwise specified 124
Atypical. *See* Psychotic disorder not otherwise specified 124
Shared. *See* Induced psychotic disorder 123

Paranoid personality disorder 189

Paranoid type, Schizophrenia 118

Paraphilias 161
Exhibitionism 161
Fetishism 161
Frotteurism 162
not otherwise specified 164
Pedophilia 162
Sexual masochism 163
Sexual sadism 163
Transvestic fetishism 163

    Voyeurism   164
Parasomnias   175
    Dream anxiety disorder (Nightmare disorder)   175
    not otherwise specified   176
    Sleep terror disorder   175
    Sleepwalking disorder   176
Partialism. *See* Paraphilia not otherwise spec-
        ified   164
Parent-child problem   207
Passive aggressive personality disorder   200
Pathologic intoxication. *See* Idiosyncratic alcohol
        intoxication   87
Pathological gambling   180
Pavor Nocturus. *See* Sleep terror disorder   175
Pedophilia   162
Persecutory type, Delusional (paranoid) disor-
        der   120
Personality disorders   189
    Antisocial   193
    Avoidant   197
    Borderline   196
    Dependent   198
    Histrionic   192
    Multiple   157
    Narcissistic   192
    not otherwise specified   200
    Obsessive compulsive   199
    Organic   105
    Paranoid   189
    Passive aggressive   200
    Sadistic   214
    Schizoid   190
    Schizotypal   191
    Self-defeating   216
Pervasive developmental disorders   49
    Autistic disorder   49
    not otherwise specified   52

Phase of life problem or other life circumstance
    problem 207
Phencyclidine (PCP) or similarly acting arylcyclohex-
    ylamine use disorders, abuse/dependence 110
Phencyclidine (PCP) or similarly acting arylcyclo-
    hexylamine-induced organic mental disor-
    ders 98
  delirium 99
  delusional disorder 100
  intoxication 98
  mixed organic mental disorder. *See* Phencyclidine
    (PCP) or similarly acting arlycyclohexlyamine-
    induced organic mental disorder not otherwise
    specified 100
  mood disorder 100
  organic mental disorder not otherwise spec-
    ified 100
Phobia
  Simple 144
  Social 143
Physical complaints. *See* Adjustment disorder with
    physical complaints 185
Physical condition, Psychological factors affect-
    ing 187
Pica 64
Pick's disease. *See* Presenile dementia not otherwise
    specified 86
Polysubstance dependence 110
Post-traumatic stress disorder 146
Posthallucinogen perception disorder 95
Premature ejaculation 167
Premenstrual syndrome. *See* Late luteal phase dys-
    phoric disorder 213
Presenile dementia. *See* Primary degenerative de-
    mentia of the Alzheimer type, presenile
    onset 85 or Presenile dementia not otherwise
    specified 86

not otherwise specified 86

Primary degenerative dementia of the Alzheimer type 84

Primary hypersomnia 173

Primary insomnia 172

Profound mental retardation 48

Pseudocyesis. *See* Conversion disorder 151

Pseudodementia. *See* Major depressive episode 128 or Dementia 78

Pseudoneurotic schizophrenia. *See* Schizotypal personality disorder 191

Pseudopsychosis. *See* Factitious disorder with psychological symptoms 177

Psychoactive substance abuse 109

Psychoactive substance abuse not otherwise specified 111

Psychoactive substance dependence 107

Psychoactive substance dependence not otherwise specified 111

Psychoactive substance use disorders (by substance) 107

  Alcohol 109

  Amphetamine or similarly acting sympathomimetic 109

  Cannabis 109

  Cocaine 110

  Hallucinogen 110

  Inhalant 110

  Nicotine 110

  Opioid 110

  Phencyclidine (PCP) or similarly acting arylcyclohexylamine 110

  Sedative, hypnotic, or anxiolytic 110

Psychoactive substance-induced organic mental disorders (by substance) 86

  Alcohol 86

  Amphetamine or similarly acting sympathomimetic 89

Caffeine 91
Cannabis 91
Cocaine 92
Hallucinogen 94
Inhalant 96
Nicotine 97
Opioid 97
Other or unspecific psychoactive substance 103
Phencyclidine (PCP) or similarly acting arylcyclo-
hexylamine 98
Sedative, hypnotic, or anxiolytic 101
Psychogenic
amnesia 157
fugue 157
pain disorder. *See* Somatoform pain disorder 155
Psychological factors affecting physical condi-
tion 187
Psychosexual dysfunctions. *See* Sexual dysfunc-
tions 164
Psychosexual disorder not elsewhere classified. *See*
Sexual disorder not elsewhere specified 168
Psychosis with Cerebral Arteriosclerosis. *See* Multi-
infarct dementia 85
Psychotic depressive reaction. *See* Major depres-
sion 135
Psychotic disorders
Brief reactive psychosis 121
Delusional (paranoid) disorder 119
Induced psychotic disorder 123
Major depressive episode with psychotic fea-
tures 130
Manic episode with psychotic features 127
not otherwise specified 124
Organic delusional disorder 105
Organic hallucinosis 81
Schizoaffecive disorder 123
Schizophrenia 113
Schizophreniform disorder 122

Psychotic disorders not elsewhere classified   121
   Brief reactive psychosis   121
   Induced psychotic disorder   123
   Psychotic disorder not otherwise specified   124
   Schizoaffective disorder   123
   Schizophreniform disorder   122
Pyromania   180

Rapid cycling. *See* Bipolar disorder, mixed   132
Reactive attachment disorder of infancy and early
   childhood   73
Reading disorder. *See* Developmental reading disor-
   der   53
Receptive language disorder. *See* Developmental
   receptive language disorder   54
Residual type, Schizophrenia   118
Retardation, Mental   47
Rum fits. *See* Alcohol withdrawal delirium 88 or
   Uncomplicated alcohol withdrawal   87
Rumination disorder of infancy   65

Sadistic personality disorder   214
Scatalogia, Telephone. *See* Paraphilia not otherwise
   specified   164
Schizoaffective disorder   123
Schizoid disorder of childhood or adolescence. *See*
   Pervasive development disorders   49
Schizoid personality disorder   190
Schizophrenia   113
   catatonic type   117
   disorganized type   117
   paranoid type   118
   residual type   118
   undifferentiated type   118
Schizophrenic disorders. *See* Schizophrenia   113
Schizophreniform disorder   122
Schizotypal personality disorder   191
School phobia. *See* Separation anxiety disorder   61

Seasonal depression. *See* Major depression, seasonal pattern 131

Seasonal mood disorders. *See* Mood disorders, seasonal pattern 131

Sedative, hypnotic, or anxiolytic use disorders, abuse/dependence 110

Sedative, hypnotic, or anxiolytic-induced organic mental disorders 101
  amnestic disorder 103
  intoxication 101
  Uncomplicated, withdrawal 101
  withdrawal delirium 102

Senile dementia. *See* Primary degenerative dementia of the Alzheimer type, senile onset 84 or Senile dementia not otherwise specified 86
  not otherwise specified 86

Separation anxiety disorder 61

Severe mental retardation 48

Sexual arousal disorder 165
  Female sexual arousal disorder 165
  Male sexual arousal disorder. *See* Male erectile disorder 166

Sexual aversion disorder 165

Sexual desire disorders 165
  Hypoactive sexual desire disorder 165
  Sexual aversion disorder 165

Sexual deviations. *See* Paraphilias 161

Sexual disorders 161
  not otherwise specified 168
  Paraphilias 161
  Sexual dysfunctions 164

Sexual dysfunctions 164
  not otherwise specified 168
  Orgasm disorders 166
  Sexual arousal disorders 165
  Sexual desire disorders 165
  Sexual pain disorders 167

Sexual masochism   163
Sexual pain disorders   167
   Dyspareunia   167
   Vaginismus   168
Sexual sadism   163
Shared paranoid disorder. *See* Induced psychotic
      disorder   123
Simple phobia   144
Simple schizophrenia. *See* Schizotypal personality
      disorder   191
Sleep disorders   171
   Dyssomnias   171
   Parasomnias   175
Sleep terror disorder   175
Sleep-wake schedule disorder   174
Sleepwalking disorder   176
Social phobia   143
Socialized conduct disorder, Aggressive/Nonag-
      gressive. *See* Conduct disorder, group type   59
Sociopathic personality. *See* Antisocial personality
      disorder   193
Solitary aggressive type, conduct disorder. *See* Con-
      duct disorder, solitary aggressive type   59
Somatic type, Delusional (paranoid) disorder   120
Somatization disorder   153
Somatoform disorders   151
   Body dysmorphic disorder   151
   Conversion disorder   151
   Hypochondriasis   152
   not otherwise specified   156
   Somatization disorder   153
   Somatoform pain disorder   155
   Undifferentiated somatoform disorder   155
Somatoform pain disorder   155
Somnambulism. *See* Sleepwalking disorder   176
Specific developmental disorders   52
   Academic skills disorder   52

Language and speech disorders 53
Motor skills disorder 55
not otherwise specified 55
Specific phobias. *See* Simple phobia 144
Speech disorders, developmental. *See* Language
and speech disorders (developmental) 53
Speech disorders not elsewhere classified 72
Cluttering 72
Stuttering 72
Speed. *See* Amphetamine or other similarly acting
sympathomimetic
Stereotyped movement disorders. *See* Stereotypy/
habit disorder 74 or Tic disorders 68
Stereotypy/habit disorder 74
Stress disorder, Post-traumatic. *See* Post-traumatic
stress disorder 146
Stuttering 72
Substance use. *See* Psychoactive substance use
Substance-induced organic mental disorders. *See*
Psychoactive substance-induced organic mental
disorders 86
Symbiotic psychosis. *See* Pervasive developmental
disorders 49
Sympathomimetic. *See* Amphetamine or similiarly
acting sympathomimetic

THC. *See* Cannabis
Tic disorders 68
Chronic motor or vocal tic disorder 69
not otherwise specified 70
Tourette's disorder 69
Transient tic disorder 70
Tobacco. *See* Nicotine
Tourette's disorder 69
Transient tic disorder 70
Transsexualism 67
Transvestic fetishism 163

Transvestism. *See* Transvestic fetishism   163
Traumatic neurosis. *See* Post-traumatic stress disor-
      der   146
Trichotillomania   181

Uncomplicated alcohol withdrawal   87
Uncomplicated bereavement   208
Uncomplicated sedative, hypnotic, or anxiolytic
      withdrawal   101
Undersocialized conduct disorder. *See* Conduct dis-
      order   58
   Aggressive type. *See* Conduct disorder, solitary
      aggressive type   59
   Nonaggressive type. *See* Conduct disorder, un-
      differentiated type   59
Undifferentiated attention-deficit disorder   74
Undifferentiated somatoform disorder   155
Undifferentiated type, Schizophrenia   118
Unspecified mental disorder (nonpsychotic)   209
Unspecified mental retardation   48
Unspecified substance dependence. *See* Psychoac-
      tive substance dependence not otherwise spec-
      ified   111
Urophilia. *See* Paraphilia not otherwise spec-
      ified   164

Vaginismus   168
Vocal, Chronic motor or, tic disorder. *See* Chronic
      motor or vocal tic disorder   69
Voyeurism   164

Withdrawal. *See* Adjustment disorder with with-
      drawal   185
Withdrawal   81
   Alcohol, Uncomplicated   87
   Amphetamine or similarly acting sym-
      pathomimetic   89

    Cocaine 97
    Nicotine 97
    Opioid 98
    Other or unspecified psychoactive substance 103
    Sedative, hypnotic, or anxiolytic, Uncompli-
      cated 101
  Withdrawal delirum
    Alcohol 88
    Sedative, hypnotic, or anxiolytic 102
  Work inhibition. _See_ Adjustment disorder with work
    (or academic) inhibition 185
  Writing disorder. _See_ Developmental expressive
    writing disorder 52

  Zoophilia. _See_ Paraphilia not otherwise spec-
    ified 164